EXPIRATION DATE

Sergiu Damian

NO EXPIRATION DATE

SIMPLE, EASY-TO-FOLLOW RULES TO
LIVING WELL AT 100 AND BEYOND

Volume 1

Damian, Sergiu
No Expiration Date
Simple, Easy-to-Follow Rules to
Living Well at 100 and Beyond
Copyright © Sergiu Damian 2014

E-mail address:
noexpirationdate1@gmail.com

Table of Contents

This book is dedicated to all those who want to stay young, beautiful and healthy until the end of their days.

Foreword

Better to die young at 120 years old than to die old at 70.
Sergiu Damian

Many people, young and old, ask themselves how they might stay healthy and live a long life. Thus we wonder what choices we should make in order to safeguard our health and extend our lives as long as possible.

When I first read Sergiu Damian's book, I was really surprised. I could not believe that he managed to gather, in one single book, so much important advice that is useful for living longer.

I met the author in 2001 at a party. There he gave a speech on a number of nutritional deficiencies where he determined that there is a situation of deep imbalance in the health of many individuals.

In this series of volumes—of easy and immediate comprehension—one of the highest experts on longevity will explain how to reach 120 years of age. The good news is that this is not the usual book that says the same things dictated by passing trends—the typical mixture of true and false theories which are hardly distinguishable one from another. In fact, it was written precisely to "separate the wheat from the chaff," namely, to separate the right theories from the wrong ones that are hidden among them.

I could say that Sergiu Damian is one of the best experts on longevity, but that would not be enough; this author is a visionary of health, an exceptional teacher, and a professional who is always up to date.

His book is the most accessible guide to the comprehension of the basic principles of health that I have ever seen. The key to well-being lies in distinguishing theories which are true from those that are false; it is not about diets, nutritional supplements, or sports. Rather, it is about following a correct lifestyle, a set of principles that we will discover later in the book.

Reading this book should be compulsory for every person who really cares about his or her health, not to mention the many professional men and women who need it. What at first glance seems to be a normal guide about health is, in reality, one of the few books in the world that deals effectively with the secrets of youth and beauty.

We are constantly overwhelmed with books that promise health and well-being, volumes which often are not worth reading. If a reader finds a book that says salt has to be used in moderation, throw it out the window! Salt is always bad, even when used in small quantities. The same thing goes for coffee and sugar.

At home, Sergiu has a library that has more than 4,000 books about health, well-being, longevity, as well as philosophy, computer science, mathematics, and economics.

The thing that struck me most in the books on health I have read so far is how modern medicine and the pharmaceutical industry have been able to infiltrate and distort many irrefutable truths on the psychophysical well-being of our bodies. An example of this is the recommendation to avoid the sun, a subject on which the author tries to shed light in his first volume. In addition, I noticed that older works are less spoiled by erroneous theories than the recent versions.

Today, the literature of welfare is a morass of vague information, wrong and confusing. The information that really matters is scarce, to say the least. As if that were not enough, doctors use complicated language to refer to concepts that are not so hard to understand if they are explained in simple words. Many physicians and doctors prefer, however, to confuse the ideas and to accentuate our dependence on their services instead of offering us authentic teachings.

This book, however, will not only teach each reader; it will transform readers into persons in charge of their own health. The text contains plenty of advice; it is an intelligent teaching of the basic principles of health that goes beyond the practice of proper nutrition. That is because its purpose is still mainly to let people know about the concepts that really matter and that have been hidden from the general public.

If everyone was aware of these secrets, and I say secrets because for years they have been intentionally hidden, manipulated, or distorted, more people would live beyond one hundred years in good health. In other words, life expectancy would double.

Despite the complexity of this topic, the book is written in simple language and is easily understood. It is not a detached text full of abstract science; it is a book that meets the readers where they are.

I want to point out that the teachings you will find in this series of volumes represent some of the most important discoveries of all time about extending life. It is knowledge handed down over the centuries by the greatest minds in history that since has been hidden by modern medicine and by pharmaceutical companies.

Giacomo Rizzoli
Dietician and Nutritionist

Introduction

Diseases that afflict man, fruit of civilization, arise mainly from nutrition and, therefore, can be cured only through a proper diet.

Dr. H. P. Rusch

Another book on health, you think. There are already so many. After all, for those who want to acquire knowledge about health, or improve the health of those who already have it, or who want to take their destiny into their own hands without the help of others, it is sufficient to walk into a bookstore and head toward the *Health and Well-being* section.

But is it really so easy to find what we actually need? After carrying out an investigation, I discovered that the majority of books dealing with this subject are not serious works or are of poor quality that boast the merits of miraculous diets or try to entice the potential reader with headlines like *Elixir of Life* or *How to Live a Hundred Years*.

When we buy a house, typically we already have a basic understanding of what we should expect: if the architect is bad or dishonest, it is very likely that we will realize this.

But when it comes to health, people seem to have blind faith in their doctor or in the books they read. Why accept ignorance about health?

The main purpose of this series of volumes is to provide readers with information about the basic principles of health, wellness, and longevity.

At first I wrote this work just for me and, at most, to give copies to my family and friends. It was basically a collection of notes and reminders that, after long and careful research, I considered essential and fundamental to well-being.

My first notes date back to when I was 14 years old, when my older sister, Natalie, went to university to study medicine. Unlike my expectations, almost everything that was taught on nutrition contradicted my fragile knowledge of the time. In fact, my sister and I often quarreled on the subject. Oddly enough, my parents always agreed with her.

When after years of research and experience my theories began to prove true, all my relatives and friends asked me to write a book. The simple rules in this and the next volume have worked wonders on me and on thousands of others who have put them into practice.

EXPERIENCE COUNTS

For 25 years I have been studying and experimenting[1] with the theories of the greatest nutritionists on Earth, from American researchers to Russian, European, Chinese, and Japanese.

Among the different research I studied, I was impressed particularly by one of the latest discoveries about the lifespan of humans and animals. Some recent studies have shown that human life has no age limit and is in constant evolution.

---

1 I experimented with various diets on me and I monitored those of others.

Experiments on various animals, in fact, showed a lengthening of 50–75 percent in the average life of each animal. As we will see later, this figure is likely to grow further.

But this is not an absolute novelty because cases of extreme longevity have occurred in the past. There is no religion or culture in the world that does not speak of people who have lived more than 200 years.

Although there is no evidence in this regard, scientists share the view that this kind of longevity isn't impossible.

WHO AM I?

Probably, at this moment, some readers will be wondering if I'm a researcher, a scientist, a doctor, or something similar. Well, not really. I have studied all these specialties by myself without the help of universities. I am, in fact, a nutritionist and self-taught researcher.[2]

The thought of eternal youth has fascinated me since childhood. At eight years of age, I had already studied the religions of the world together with their doctrines. I liked science and wanted to assimilate all the knowledge in the world.

I was always looking for answers: why we die, why some of us live longer than others, and why some people age faster than others, and so on.

---

2 In fact this is an advantage and security for the reader, as the author has no secondary interests that may interfere with those of the reader. For example, physicians who do not comply with the doctrines of modern medicine and the pharmaceutical industry are likely to be mocked and therefore jeopardize their careers. When we are "inside" we must defend the interests of the group. The thing is simple: the sick are the "raw material" of doctors. If patients no longer existed, doctors and the pharmaceutical multinationals would starve or change jobs.

When I was growing up, I wanted to be many things: a scientist, an astronaut, an oceanographer, a circus performer, or a musician. But the "profession" that attracted me more than anything else was "to live a long time without getting old."

When my older sister went to university to study medicine, her choice strengthened my interest in health even more. So the thought of longevity entered my field of study and absorbed all my attention. When I was 14, I had a very specific purpose—to discover the secrets of life. Since then, these studies continue to be my main goal.

THE UNIVERSITY AND ITS HALF-TRUTHS

About 25 years ago I began my career as an independent researcher. I began to put into practice some of the theories presented in this book. One of the first things I did was remove salt and its derivatives from my diet, including those hidden in foods.

My sister was really worried about me because I did not eat salt for a year. In fact, at the university she was taught that human beings should include cooking salt in their diet. She told me that if I did not immediately reinstate salt in my diet, in a short time I would lose all my body fluids, my mouth and my throat would be dry, and I would become ill. For her it was a miracle that I was still alive.[3]

---

3 Sodium—together with potassium—helps the body maintain the correct osmotic pressure between the cells (the fluid distribution between the inside and outside of the cell) and participates in the hydro-regulation of our body. When there is too much sodium, it leads to water retention. Too little sodium leads to dehydration, just what my sister was afraid would happen to me. But our bodies do not need the sodium that is found in table salt but rather that which is found naturally in fruits and vegetables. The first is inorganic, whereas the second is organic.

Thanks to the many books concerning food research that I had read, I was already aware of those urban legends about the need for salt, so I tried not to be influenced and remained firm in my beliefs.

At first, none of my family members would listen to me. Everything my sister said was law for them. In fact, she was about to become a doctor.

Today, I am 40 years old, but I look much younger. I have never used any cream for wrinkles, tablets, elixirs, or something to keep me young looking, nor have I suffered from any disease.

Every now and then, when I go to the hospital to have a checkup, the doctors tell me I have the internal organs comparable to those of a child.

Many, who do not know my age, even if they are 10–15 years younger than me, think I'm younger than they are. They cannot believe my age even when I show an identity document. They remain perplexed and incredulous.

THE END OF THE STORY

Here is how the story with my sister ended. After studying six years at the university, she took her first degree. After another four years she completed her specialization. During her studies she won several competitions and obtained various diplomas. Then she went to work at the Military Hospital in the capital of our country. It had been 15 years since that conversation on salt when one day my sister came to me desperately.

"You know, Sergiu," she said, "I'm worried about my health. So far I have never spoken to you about it."

"What happened to you?" I asked.

"I have very high blood pressure." And she began to tell me her problem.

I must confess that I already knew about her problems from our mother, but I decided not to intervene; after all, she was a doctor. I knew that her pride in being a doctor would not allow her to ask me even for an opinion, at least for a while.

Her problem had appeared five years before that conversation, when she was 32 years old. Despite all the medicines she had taken, the situation continued to deteriorate. The tablets she had taken for years for petty reasons, together with the most recent ones for hypertension, had damaged her stomach and liver. Hereafter she had to add more of them to treat her stomach and liver and then take other pills for her kidneys.

So instead of getting better, she was sinking even deeper. Moreover, her headaches became an inseparable "friend." She had entered
a very dangerous downward spiral. I listened to her carefully for about five minutes without interrupting.

"What do you think?" she asked me after she finished her story.

"Do you remember when you told me to reinstate the consumption of salt?" I asked.

"I remember as if it was yesterday."

"Well, it was the salt that has caused your disease." She was aware that the medicines had caused her more harm than good.

"Do not worry; you will get well soon," I said.

"Are you saying to me that I will return to being as healthy as before?"

"It is extraordinarily simple to regain and maintain health; this is why many do not realize it."

"I'll do anything to regain my health."

Then I smiled and asked, "Tell me first where your medical theories have gone."

"I've lost them along the way," she said with a smile.

"So you're ready to abandon the old rules?"

"Sure, and now I would like to try your method," she said. "How can you teach it to me?"

"I wrote a guide on the subject. There you will find all the answers you need."

After reading the guide and putting it into practice, my sister has recovered completely. As I mentioned previously, during my journey I have helped many people who, because of misinformation, were suffering from various diseases.

As we saw in the example of my sister, doctors themselves can be victims of their own theories, and these cases unfortunately abound.

THE INDIGENOUS PEOPLE OF OUR DAYS

Noting that on average doctors live shorter lives than other people, I realized very quickly that many doctors are victims of "miraculous pills." Yet we are all responsible for our own health and there is no need to go and look for it elsewhere.

Without realizing it, we act like the American Indians when

they met Europeans for the first time. The natives used to exchange precious gold and silver for small pieces of colored glass, bronze bells, mirrors, and other things of little value. The metaphor is the following: gold and silver represent our health, whereas the pieces of colored glass and bells represent medicines and pills. Without realizing it, when we take medicines, in return we give away our health, which is much more valuable and important.

In these volumes I will present the results of the implementation of scientific research on extending life, to which I have added my own experiences.

Of course, there are plenty of books on how to take care of our health. However, this work contains something different because it represents something completely new, namely, the knowledge that is usually hidden to the general public.

IT IS NEVER TOO LATE

Some people might think that they are too young to start or too old to learn. This is a limiting belief, as a psychologist would say. Such reasoning is not only counterproductive but also brings great suffering in the future if we don't take action immediately.

Think of the diseases that some of us may be nurturing right now without even realizing it. And that is not all. Think of the suffering that those who love us and those around us might suffer, not to mention the time lost and all the money spent on medicines, which in turn might cause other diseases.

On the one hand, medicines kill us; on the other hand, they do not let us die. With this book, I undertake to offer a step-by-step guide along the path to wellness. It may seem unbelievable, but I assure you that it is feasible and that many others have already started, and they are still continuing with great results. It is never too late to begin.

AFTER THE HEALING

In 2010, when we were gathered together at a family party, my sister told all the guests how she was cured with a few simple rules after five years of trying in vain. After the party, together with a group of friends, we talked a lot about the food misinformation conveyed by modern medicine. Yet the global pharmaceutical profits in 2009 amounted to $600 billion, and by the year 2020 they will double.

Often while walking down the street we may come across "living dead persons." The pharmaceutical medicine first kills us and then, after that, it tries to keep us alive for as long as possible. And then we hear them talk about extending life.

Some people are attached to machines for 20 years in a vegetative state. Is this what we want?

THE IDEA OF THE BOOK

At the party that I mentioned above, the conversation went on until two in the morning.

"Why don't you write a book?" my sister asked. "You've done so much research during all these years. If people followed this simple advice, they would no longer need medication and a small hospital would be enough for a large city, more for injuries than for anything else. It would be a more beautiful world without all these hospitals and pharmacies. Probably there is no need even for pharmacies around the city; one would be enough for any hospital. In addition, all these trillions of dollars could be invested in other sectors. People would do something else instead of suffering from diseases. In short, it would become a different world, a better world."

"True," I said to Natalia. "I know you're right, but it is not so easy. All the people I have helped have told me the same thing. However, if I publish my book today, tomorrow will come out a thousand others that refute my theories. There is too much money at stake, and ignorance has become the queen of our time. Nowadays, in order to change a light bulb, people prefer to call the electrician and pay for that help. For health, it is the same. When we have an itchy finger, we run to the emergency room. When it comes to their own health, people trust more in others than in themselves."

My family and friends continued to urge me to write a book. Whenever I met them they would always ask, "So, did you write the book?"

THE DOUBTS

I knew it would not be an easy undertaking. I should have organized my ideas better because they were very fragmented, not to mention that I had no idea about how to write a book. In the beginning I thought that I would have to wait for another hundred years to prove to the world the validity of my theories even though people told me that my appearance and my health were the perfect demonstration. However, I let several years pass before writing the book.

During all those years, I meditated for a long time on the worrying global growth of health spending, which, in other words, means a further increase in taxes, which are already skyrocketing. To cope with the increasing number of patients, governments will have to build more hospitals, pharmacies, and emergency rooms where it will be necessary to increase medical staff.

We will come to the point in which the state cannot guarantee healthcare to everyone, and those most at risk are the elderly and the unemployed. People believe, or still hope, that the state can solve health and economic problems exactly when its ability to act is decreasing and health problems are increasing.

THE BEGINNING OF A NEW ERA

Since the fall of the Berlin Wall in 1989, and the birth of the World Wide Web in 1991, the face of the world has changed. This period, rather than marking the failure of communism, marked the end of the Industrial Age and the beginning of the Information Technology Age. Such change has already threatened the financial and health security of hundreds of millions of people, most of whom are not yet aware of the consequences.

Today politicians do not hold the power, as it was during the Industrial Age. Many people still have a mindset focused on the rights guaranteed by the large state apparatus and large companies of the Industrial Age.

The state will find itself more and more forced to unload health costs on the shoulders of its citizens. In other words, if you have money, take care of yourself; otherwise you will have to handle the costs some other way. For this reason, I believe that now more than ever we need a new culture of health and well-being that focuses on a healthy diet.

THE DOUBTS CONTINUE

Another "problem" that I was worried about was that my not having studied at the university would cause most people to not believe me or not trust me.

I know that many people are sure that everything modern medicine says is law. But I do not think it is. When I was little, I had my own way of distinguishing the theories, methods, and diets that were effective from those that were ineffective. I only needed to look at the physiques and the faces of those who held those theories.

If I saw that the doctors or experts in question were slender and appeared to be several years younger than their real age, then I knew that they were telling the truth. Conversely, if they were overweight, tired, full of wrinkles, and looking older than they really were, then I would know I had to stay away from their theories.

Today in the advertising of beauty products we see only girls and boys aged from 18 to 24. I would rather see those who produce the creams. Are they so young and without cellulite too? For many, advertising has almost become a medical prescription.

Nowadays, there are many people who follow precisely all the false pronouncements of doctors. But the most dangerous ones are the hundreds of diets and treatments that have appeared recently, their creators taking advantage of people's confidence.

120 YEARS AND BEYOND

There are people who have lived well beyond the age of 120 years. For example, Shirali Muslumov and Mahmud Eyvazov from Azerbaijan arrived at the beautiful age of 168 and 152 years respectively.

If that were not enough, I can also name the Chinese herbalist Li Ching-Yuen, who lived 256 years, according to other sources, 197 years ago. The story of Li appeared, with his obituary, in *The New York Times* on May 6, 1933.

With the advent of the computer age, we have more and more reports of long-lived people discovered by chance in the most remote places.

This is the case of the Turkish grandmother Halime Olcay, 135 years of age and still alive in 2009. So even though this book is about how to live to 120 years, a person could get up to 135 years or more. In this book, in order not to frighten the readers or arouse their suspicion, I prefer to indicate a figure that is more "credible."

WHOM TO BELIEVE?

Unfortunately, today people do not know whom to trust, whom to believe, whom not to, and what books to refer to. The market is invaded by thousands of guides and books on health, some more publicized than others. All this has become a real business, but this is not the problem. The real problems are the opposing theories of these books. In other words, the theories according to one book appear to be fine, but then, according to another book, are instead harmful.

Every day new "miraculous" therapies are invented. All the while valid textbooks are completely missing. Furthermore, they are not even advertised. Why? The answer is simple— similar books do not yield huge gains and, indeed, would collapse many industries.

A LEOPARD CANNOT CHANGE ITS SPOTS

Many who read again books on health and well-being that they have previously read, will find that what they thought was healthy before is now harmful, and what was harmful now favors good health.

An inexperienced reader in medicine might feel very confused. After all, I was feeling the same at the beginning. It took me several years of study, research, and observations before distinguishing the true ways of health.

Why is the content of the texts in question constantly changing? It is simple: some want to confuse the ideas and guide people on the wrong paths. If they would tell the truth, people would no longer need pills and doctors. It would be sufficient just to have a single book for life, a kind of bible for health; instead, they are perpetrating a false search for people and are forcing them to buy a new book every year to "stay uninformed" with great benefits for the industries that sponsor those books.

The result: the contents of the books change, but not their aim; they lead us into error.

WHOSE FAULT IS IT?

When we become ill, we are good at blaming others, starting with the pharmaceutical industry and continuing to the food industry and then the chemical industries.[4] We point the finger at them because through medicines, food colorants, and preservatives that are produced or used, we become slaves of disease and die prematurely.

Certainly this is not a problem for the pharmaceutical companies. On the contrary, these industries earn billions of dollars

---

4 People, after they are ill, become more aware of their mistakes.

and even pay taxes; otherwise they could not exist. We must not forget that first they are businesses, which by their nature are profit-making and, as such, are just doing their duty.

On the other hand, we do not have to complain about the pollution of water, land, and air. In one way or another, we ourselves contribute to the pollution of the planet or destroy each other.

We know very well that the law of supply and demand regulates the market. Who would ever invest in a business without profits?

If people took better care of their health—instead of delegating it to others—they certainly would not buy all these poisons that are sold in the pharmacies. It is so true that the word drug comes from the Greek word *pharmakon*, which, in addition to remedy, also means poison.

The root of the problem is not industries or even misleading books, but it is us or, even more, our mentality. In our ignorance, we feed these poisonous sectors. If there were no demand, none would be offered. We are the ones who hurt ourselves, despite the fact that we do not realize it. The only way to safeguard the world's health, which is a slave of the pharmaceutical companies, is to increase the information about pharmaceutical products.

THE WORLD HAS CHANGED ITS SHAPE BUT NOT ITS ESSENCE

In the film by Iovita Vlad, *The Horse, the Gun, and the Wife* (Calul, Puca și Nevasta, USSR, 1975), inspired by popular Moldavian legends about the courageous haiducs[5] guided by Novac Gruia in the fight of the peasants against the Turkish occupants (18th century), the hero said, "In life there are three things you should not entrust to anybody: your horse, your gun, and your wife."

Taking into account some aspects of the film, I noticed that the world has not changed that much since then in its struggle for survival. If people perished by the sword back then, today they die from drugs and bad food.

Today we can compare the gun to the mind because with it we will defend ourselves against crooks and health predators. At that time, holding a rifle in one's hands was safer than giving it to someone else because most of the time other people turned out to be enemies. Similarly, the same could happen today when we trust someone else with our health.

For this reason, today more than ever we must learn how to use the gun of our minds. There are sharks in all oceans, so there will always be someone ready to take advantage of us in any life context, be it health, finances, or anything else. That is why I say we should keep the gun of our minds loaded and not entrust it to others.

If I go into a store and ask the saleswoman for advice on a product I want to buy, she will probably recommend the item that they sell the least. Like all sellers, she will try to sell me the product that cannot be sold; traders love the kind of customer who can be talked into buying a product.

We can compare the horse to health. If I take good care of it,

5 In Romanian "haiduc" indicated each of the Balkan organized rebels against the Turkish domain.

the animal will be more robust, healthy, and strong, which will then take me further along the road of life. But, at the same time, I must also protect it from wolves and jackals. I use the gun that is my mind.

I always say, a hundred small steps are better than a giant one. Better to have a little knowledge in all branches than to be specialized in one, which most of the time is the purpose of our professions. What does this mean? It's simple; if I want to be healthy and live a long time, I should study health. If I want to be rich, I should study economics and finance, and so on. But I should not wait for someone else to do it for me.

WHO LOSES HIS LIFE?

While the majority of industries contribute to sustaining and improving our lives, there are a few that tend to do the exact opposite. This does not mean that the chemical, pharmaceutical, agricultural, and food industries are always dangerous, but on average the damage they create far outweighs the benefits.

For example, in the chemical industry, in spite of the great strides made in the creation of new products and compounds, there are still many companies that continue to use hundreds of harmful substances. Of the approximately 83,000 chemical products in commerce, only a hundred can be considered environmentally friendly. Others accumulate in the human body and in nature creating serious environmental damage and diseases such as cancer. In the case of some products, we do not even know the risks or the information relating to them that is contradictory.

Meanwhile our land and food are saturated with chemicals

and we keep trying to stay healthy. Modern medicine, although it has brought us numerous advantages, has also made us drug addicts.

Since the end of World War II, the production of synthetic drugs has led to an enormous development of the pharmaceutical industry, and its sales have reached astronomical levels in the world. So today these products are more a way to make money than to fight diseases. As a matter of fact, large amounts of money are spent to invent new medicines and to promote sales with expensive advertising campaigns in order to secure a slice of the lucrative market.

Therefore, today not only physicians but also patients have come to the point of putting all their trust in chemotherapy; too many people believe that synthetic drugs, or chemotherapeutic ones, are the only drugs that can achieve some results.

Look at the food industry. Whether we like it or not, we live in the age of supermarkets. Every year the average consumer spends the equivalent of two working weeks pushing a cart, and at the end of the year has carried several tons of goods purchased after appropriate selection.

But what exactly ends up every week in our shopping carts? Most of all, processed foods, i.e., foods subjected to some kind of transformation before arriving on the shelves of the supermarket.

Food can actually be bleached, colored, flavored, stabilized, vacuum packed, heat-sealed, wrapped in cellophane, canned, frozen, and, in some countries, even treated with radiation. If we compare the ingredients of these products with the products we buy, they are totally different in terms of taste, aroma, consistency, and nutritional value.

At each stage of the food's journey to our stomachs, unwelcome transformations are made. The longer the processing chain through which food passes before ending up in the hands of the consumer, the greater the need to store it and to give it better color and flavor—through the use of large amounts of chemicals.

Food industries, those that deal with the massive transformation of food, are in love with words and phrases like "convenience," "great choice," and "to meet the demand of the public," when they have to be accountable for their activities. But the hard truth is that the primary purpose of food processing is company profit.

In short, everyone gains except the people who pay with their lives. It is about economic interests. Making a profit is more important than our lives. Many hundreds of billions of euros are at stake, to the unfortunate detriment of human health.

Often people are forced to spend their life savings on hospitals, diseases, and sleepless nights full of pain, and no one is interested in helping them.

With this guide, and those that will follow, you will know how to defend yourself from junk books that lead you straight into the traps of the profiteers. Moreover, you will learn what to do to have a healthy life and, especially, how to cross the threshold of one hundred years in good health.

Everything shown in these volumes cannot be understood immediately. This is why both those who enjoy good health and those who are sick should read them several times for protection from future suffering.

THE MANY BENEFITS

Our purpose is the following: to live more than a hundred years in good health, which is not a small thing. Remember that human life can easily reach up to 130 years, and some people say that it could reach 200 years.

But since no one has officially arrived at this age yet, there is nothing left for us but waiting. Who knows, maybe it can happen that a reader of this book will achieve that goal.

I really hope it happens. But what will really change in a person's life after reading this book? What does this book offer? There are many benefits. First of all, a person will not feel tired anymore. He will always be in fine shape without following any particular therapy. He will not take any pill for losing weight because he will never put on weight. He will not have to use creams for wrinkles because his face will always be young, even when he gets "old."

Such a person will forget the word "hospital." He will not get sick anymore. He will not use medicines and he will not spend thousands of euros on therapies. (After all, sometimes even money cannot help us. Think for example, of the co-founder of Apple, Steve Jobs, who died at age 56 of a tumor in spite of a fortune of 83 billion dollars.)

Think of someone who dies at 52 because of a heart attack, or at 43 because of a tumor, and leaves a wife (or a husband) and children just when that person has reached a decent standard of living and all his loved ones need him most. Now imagine the opposite, someone who at the age of 108 or 115 years is still in good health. There is a huge difference. However, we know that a goal becomes possible only when there is someone working to achieve that goal.

Everything depends on the individual. No one should give up along the way or be misled by other manuals and theories because they only lead us astray—unless, of course, those other books reflect the content of this book. After a while, each person will understand which of the books are telling the truth and which are not.

SOME CLARIFICATIONS

After each chapter, there are two sections: *Lives of the Long-Living* and *Myth or reality?*

In the first section, *Lives of the Long-Living*, there will be a brief history that tells the extraordinary life of one of the individuals who lived more than 120 years. Some stories are longer than others, according to the information available.

It was not easy to find this information because in most cases these were people who lived in the shadows far from civilization in the most remote places of the world. In this section, in addition to the highlights, there will be some curiosities reported.

The idea of including this section stemmed from the desire to provide an extra stimulus to the reader. Besides motivating the reader, it will also help him to understand what unites all these centenarians and what we can learn directly from their experience.

In the second section, *Myth or Reality?*, the reader will be put face to face with myths and their falsehoods. In this part, through a series of examples and real-world demonstrations, many popular beliefs from the scientific world will be proved wrong.

DISCOVERING THE DEAF FLIES

Here is how a myth can become a scientific discovery. A friend of mine, a professor of a European university and an internationally-renowned researcher, told me that in the 1970s he and his colleagues were almost forced to make a scientific discovery in a fixed period of time. If my friend could not complete the task in time, he would lose his job.

We all know that making a discovery takes a long time (often years), a lot of patience, education, research, and, above all, intuition. Sometimes, despite all effort, the work does not produce the desired results.

My friend told me that some scientists were forced to draw hasty conclusions in order to relieve some of the pressure that was put on them.

The tests were not carried out to the end and, most of the time, were based on limited data and observations. This is the reason that so often drug disasters have occurred at the expense of the civilian population.

Just to give an example, read the testimony[6] of Dr. David J. Graham, a scientist with the FDA. He shared his story before the Congress of the United States on November 18, 2004.

The scientist talked about the drug Vioxx, an anti-inflammatory used all over the world. According to his research, after its first appearance in 1999 and until 2004 the drug caused between 88,000 and 139,000 heart attacks and strokes in the United States alone.

---

6 Internet website: http://www.finance.senate.gov/imo/media/doc/111804dgtest.pdf

Dr. Graham made a comparison with plane crashes. Based on an average of 150–200 people per aircraft, from 500 to 900 aircrafts should have crashed to equal the number of people who have suffered heart attacks or strokes. This means two to four aircraft accidents a week for five years.

At that time among scientists, my friend told me there was even a joke to give a better idea of the situation:

As homework, a science teacher gives her students a free experiment about the animal world. Peter goes home, sits down and thinks. Time passes, but he has no ideas at all. After two hours, a fly settles in front of him. Happy to have found the object of his search, Peter captures the fly. He carefully observes it closely, turns it and finally decides to start the experiment. He rips off its wings and orders it to fly. "Fly, fly!"

But all the fly does is scamper around on the table. So he orders it again to "Fly!" The fly is still walking. At this point Peter concludes his experiment.

Satisfied with his discovery, he opens his notebook and writes, "If we tear the wings off of a fly, it will not listen to us."

Unfortunately, in today's scientific world, there are many "discoveries" similar to that of Peter. And, to many of us, it seems that it matters very little whether it is a real discovery or a scientific illusion—hence the deaf fly. Be careful. You can no longer hope to obtain medical care by experienced and reliable professionals. The only solution is to learn to take care of yourself, and this book will teach you how.

Sergiu Damian,
August 8, 2014

37

CHAPTER 1

THE SECRET OF HIPPOCRATES

As a physician, I believe it is essential that the diet therapy is and remains the foundation of all the efforts made toward healing.

Dr. M. Gerson

It would be unfair not to start from the beginning, namely, from the founding father of medicine, Hippocrates.

The leitmotif of this book is nothing more than the secular evolution of the true teachings of the Greek doctor that were forgotten or hidden for centuries and then picked up by the early pioneers of nutritional science.

We have to consider that the father of medicine, Hippocrates, introduced the innovative concept that illness and the health of a person depend on the specific circumstances in which the person has lived. Furthermore, he was the first to study anatomy and pathology through the dissection of dead bodies.

Hippocrates became famous in ancient times when he helped overcome the great plague of Athens in 429 BC. To him we owe the importance of the concepts of diet and nutrition. Still, today, Hippocrates is considered one of the most famous physicians of all time. His motto was: "Let your food be your medicine, and medicine your food."

So the Greek doctor recommended to both healthy persons and sick ones, either to prevent diseases or to treat them, a diet of raw foods. These were natural foods, carefully chosen, which had to cleanse the body, eliminate the excess of acid, and restore vitality.

Not by chance did he always say to the sick people he visited, "We are what we eat." His secret was, in fact, eating foods that would feed and cure at the same time. Thanks to his method, Hippocrates could heal countless diseases.

Today, nutrition lacks enzymes, vitamins, mineral salts, antioxidants, and other micronutrients that are essential for our health. This leads to a progressive weakening of our bodies, promotes the onset of various diseases, and shortens life.

A REAL CASE

After we were married for some time, my wife was diagnosed with an ovarian cyst that had to be removed as soon as possible. My wife booked the surgery without letting me know, giving the excuse that she was going to visit her mother for a week.

Luckily, I found out what she intended to do the day before the surgery. So I went to the hospital in a hurry and brought her back home. Meanwhile, I told her to eat only raw food, like raw milk, raw fruits, and raw vegetables. After four months, the doctors repeated the scan. And guess what? There was not even a shadow of a cyst. The doctor who had diagnosed the cyst four months earlier could not believe his eyes. The cyst had disappeared.

Physicians today, and especially patients¬, want to obtain healing as fast as possible. Hippocrates' method, however, has the advantage of acting with safety. Immediately after the beginning of the treatment, the disease does not evolve further. For this reason, any doctor can recommend Hippocrates' method. It is harmless; it can be practiced without the fear of adverse effects and without conflicting with the instructions of modern medicine.

Raw foods nourish us and heal us at the same time. After just three weeks a person can feel the tiredness disappear and, surprisingly, the deposits of unnecessary fat disappear too. Resistance and strength grow, even under conditions of heavy work. And thirst produced by the effort decreases considerably.

Hippocrates' method, with respect to modern medicine which simply eliminates the symptoms, eliminates the cause.

SAHAN DOSOVA

Sahan Dosova (March 27, 1879–May 9, 2009) was a woman from Kazakhstan. The Kazakh super-centenarian died at the age of 130 years and 43 days after she slipped and fell on the floor of her bathroom. Her identity card and Kazakh Soviet passport confirm her date of birth. Demographers found her name in the census of Stalin in 1926 proving she was then 47 years old. This seems to confirm that her year of birth was 1879.

Sahan's parents died of plague when she was six years old. She married her first husband at the age of 17 and gave birth to eight children. During the famine in 1930 she lost her husband and also all her children. Afterwards, she married her husband's brother, according to the Kazakh tradition.

By her second husband, Sahan had three children, and they gave her 37 grandchildren and many great-grandchildren. She became a widow for the second time when her husband lost his life in the Battle of Stalingrad during World War II. The woman said she saw Lenin and Stalin.

HER SECRET

In an interview she gave in March 2009, Sahan Dosova said, "I don't have any particular secret. I have never taken pills and when I was sick I used grandma's remedies. I have never eaten sweets because I don't like them." In another interview, when she was asked to reveal her secret, she simply said, "Garlic."

The super-centenarian lady also attributed her long life to her sense of humor.

IS A GENIUS BORN OR MADE?

The first myth I want to debunk is the one that says we are born geniuses. People are not born sunny-natured or moody, brave or shy, optimistic or pessimistic. In the same way, they are not born painters, composers, or athletes. Talent does not exist *a priori*, nor does personality.

When we hear people say that a specific person is born to do one thing or another, we should know that this is not so. The good news is that we are all born as equals. Everybody at the gaming table of life has the same cards to play at the formation of the zygote (the result of the fusion between the ovum and the sperm). The following is what makes the difference: the fact that we belong to a family and a geographic area that is considered "healthy," with basic learning, studies, and experiences.

Each of us was born equal to a Mozart or an Einstein. We *become* geniuses; we are not born like that. The belief that talent, predisposition to disease, or even a long life, are transmitted by inheritance is absolutely false. To further analyze this argument, I suggest that people read the book *The Biology of Belief* by Bruce H. Lipton.[7]

Such ideas limit us and keep us from being what we want to be. Nothing has a greater impact on the unceasing process that constitutes us than the choice between optimism and pessimism. The concept of personality is overestimated. Every moment, who we are depends only on us. There is no predetermination; there are only individual choices that make us become one thing or another. We will discuss inheritance in the next volume.

According to a recent publication of the University of Cambridge, genius is not an innate gift. As a matter of fact, we need a minimum of preparation, excellent teachers, and an iron will in order to become great scientists, great musicians, or insurmountable players.

The results of this unique research are summarized in the publication by the University of Cambridge entitled *The Cambridge Handbook of Expertise and Expert Performance*, published in 2006 by *New Scientists*[8] magazine.

According to researchers at the well-known Cambridge

---

7 Lipton, B. H., March 2005. *The Biology of Belief: Unleashing the Power of Consciousness, Matter and Miracles*. USA, Santa Rosa, CA: Mountain of Love.

8 Ericsson, K. A., Charness, N., Hoffman R. R., Feltovich P. J., 2006, *The Cambridge Handbook of Expertise and Expert Performance*. Cambridge: Cambridge University Press.

University, the extraordinary abilities of individuals who are commonly considered geniuses are not innate gifts. Rather, they are the result of a skillful combination of personal qualities, education of the highest level, and hours of study and application.

Explaining how a genius is formed is not an easy matter. According to professor of psychology at Florida State University, Anders Ericsson, genius develops when an intelligent person, properly educated and supported, concentrates all his efforts on achieving skills and extraordinary competence in a particular field of human knowledge.

These individuals do not necessarily need to have an extraordinary IQ (Intelligence Quotient) but, rather, excellent teachers, an environment that will encourage them to improve continually, and, above all, a strong desire to work. And, yes, this desire is really extraordinary.

Continuous study and practice are actually a workout for the brain. Eric Kandel of Columbia University showed in one of his researches in 2000 how the continuous repetition of the same lesson increases the number and strength of nerve connections associated with our memory.[9] This research awarded him the Nobel Prize. An uninterrupted and focused study serves to build a real neural-knowledge network.

Observation of the performance of those who are considered geniuses has allowed researchers to introduce a kind of "rule of thumb." Psychologist Benjamin Bloom, of the University of Chicago, and his

---

9 Kandel, E. R., December 8, 2000. *The Molecular Biology of Memory Storage: A Dialog between Genes and Synapses*. Nobel Lecture.

colleagues, analyzed the performance of a sample of 120 illustrious personalities, including scientists, musicians, and athletes, finding that these people had worked very hard for at least ten years before being recognized as champions in their own discipline.

Mozart, for example, wrote symphonies when he was only seven years old. However, until the age of six, he had already studied 3,500 hours of music with his ambitious father, Leopold. Furthermore, he did not produce anything that made him famous before reaching adolescence. Even the greatest Olympic swimmers train an average of fifteen years before they can compete at the highest levels.

My friend Ionică Minune (Romania), who is considered the best accordion virtuoso of all time, confessed to me that he had arrived at that level not only because he started playing when he was four years old, but also because he had practiced every day for up to 18 hours. This is why Ionică has developed such an extraordinary technique, without precedent, and why he is considered a genius. He is able to compose songs directly while he is playing, just improvising. A musician graduated from a music school would spend a whole month learning such songs, without even being able to play them. But Ionică learned everything by himself, by ear, and he did not attend any music school.

Before Ionică was famous, I asked Professor Yuri Dranga, of the Moscow Conservatory, to listen to one of Ionică's songs. Professor Yuri Dranga was also an international master. His answer left me speechless, "I don't think he really plays at this speed. This is impossible. He has for sure tripled or quadrupled the speed with a tape recorder."

Hearing such words from a person of international fame made me realize the greatness of Ionică Minune who, not surprisingly, has earned the name Ionică. In Romanian Ionică stands for Johnny and Minune for Wonder. His real name is Ene Gheorghe.[10]

Another example is Zsuzsa Polgár, with her two younger sisters Judit and Zsófia, who were part of an educational program carried out by their father László Polgár. He was determined to demonstrate that a child can achieve excellent results if trained from childhood in a specific field. His motto was, "The genius is made, and does not arise alone."[11] He and his wife, Klara, educated their daughters at home, making them specialize in chess.

Also, Thomas Edison maintained that the genius is made of one percent inspiration (creativity) and 99 percent perspiration (sweat, fatigue).

We all have a thinking machine far superior to our conscious mind: the *subconscious*.[12] Mathematician John von Neumann calculated that the human brain can store up to 280 trillion bits of memory.

THE GENIUS FORMULA

Is there a formula to becoming a genius? According to the manual of Cambridge, there is. This formula is given by one percent of inspiration, 29 percent of excellent education and 70 percent of hard

---

10 Wikipedia: http://en.wikipedia.org/wiki/Ionic%C4%83_Minune

11 Flora, C., "The Grandmaster Experiment," *Psychology Today*, July 1, 2005, Internet website: http://www.psychologytoday.com/articles/200506/the-grandmaster-experiment

12 We will handle this argument in the chapter "The Power of the Mind" in the second volume.

work. There's nothing to do but to roll up our sleeves and bow down our heads in the books with the purpose of becoming the best. Will is power!

GENETIC INHERITANCE

In the next volume we will dedicate a specific chapter to genetic inheritance. There we will see how modern medicine invented the concept of inheritance and predisposition to disease either to offload its faults or for convenience.

It is not true that if my father had cancer or diabetes I run the risk of being affected by these diseases too. Neither is it true that if my parents lived about 70–80 years, I would live nearly as long as they did and would have no chance of reaching 120 years. In the same way, if my parents' lives were too short it doesn't mean that I will be like them.

In other words, science says that if, for example, the father and son both died of lung cancer, or the mother and the daughter of breast cancer, this means that both father and mother passed on the cancer to their offspring through genetic inheritance. This is not true, unless we do what we have seen them doing. But we don't want to anticipate, as we will discuss all this and more in the chapter "Inheritance" in the next volume.

CHAPTER 2

ENZYMES

*The duration of life is inversely proportional to the rate
of exhaustion of the enzymatic potential of an organism.*
Dr. E. Howell

Since the importance of vitamins for our lives was first discovered at
the beginning of the last century, science has been advertising their
relevance with a loud voice. Consequently, it was discovered that
diseases could occur due to the destruction of vitamins in cooked and
refined foods.

Why such propaganda? The reason is that vitamins can be
prepared industrially. Those who are not informed should know that
the pharmaceutical industry is one of the most profitable industrial
activities in the world. To be sure of this truth we just need to have a
look on the Internet.

WHAT HAPPENS LATER?

In 1940, American researcher Edward Howell made an important discovery. Studying some vital substances, namely *enzymes*, he showed that they are the bearers of life of any living organism—as long as they are not destroyed through cooking. Therefore, they also constitute the living matter of our foods.[13]

It is strange that science did not particularly appreciate this extraordinary discovery and that there was no advertising at all in favor of food enzymes, as happened in due course with vitamins.

Why is that so? It is very clear; enzymes are important substances that are found only in raw foods. They cannot be produced and, therefore, cannot constitute a "deal." For this reason, today we still hear more talking about vitamins than enzymes. If sick people can be cured through raw foods, without spending a penny on drugs or medical consultations, who would have an interest, apart from the sick, in disclosing that fact?

WHAT ARE ENZYMES?

Enzymes are specific proteins that contain the spark of life and maintain vegetative life in the cells of plants and animals. In nature there are different types of enzymes.

No cell division, growth, or reproduction can take place without the presence of enzymes. They are the administrators and executors that nature has placed in every living creature.

Enzymes lead chemical processes in all the organs of the

---

13 Howell, E., "Enzyme Starvation," *The Journal of the American Association for Medico-Physical Research*, III. Chicago, April 15, 1940.

human body, as well as of animals and plants. The majority of biological reactions catalyzed by enzymes have a speed millions of times superior to the speed they would have without any catalyst. The work of enzymes in our bodies is the greatest miracle of the living world.

In the human body there are two types of enzymes. One category includes the so-called ferments (endogenous enzymes), secreted by the digestive glands, which regulate digestion precisely. In the other category there are the true enzymes (exogenous), namely, those that we are interested in. The latter type of enzymes produce the reactions mentioned earlier in the organism and, particularly, contribute to cellular metabolism.

So the enormous importance of enzymes for our health is clear. They are infinitely more important than vitamins, whose function is that of auxiliary substances for the enzymes and their "couriers." Unlike the digestive ferments that the organism can produce, exogenous enzymes cannot be produced by our bodies. As the prefix "exo" shows, these catalysts must be introduced from the outside, through specific nutrition as for example, with vitamins.

All the strength and beauty that the enzymes have in a vegetable or fruit are offered to us in order to join another activity cycle, the one followed by the cells of our bodies.

This wise order represents a law of nature. The penetration of the enzymes in our cells, and the resulting bond that is formed between them, can be compared to exogamy, i.e., the entering into a family of an outsider through marriage. Then the enzyme becomes the "master of the house" and guarantees the existence and multiplication of cells. These living operators—we might say intelligent goblins—operate like real mechanical objects, controlling all the functions of the body.

WE BECOME YOUNG

The more our diet contains "fresh" enzymes, the greater the number of sources of life that pour into the body from which young cells can be formed. This means a surplus of energy and resistance and a strengthening of our immunity to diseases. It means beauty and a better functioning of glands and, consequently, better control of body weight, and also purification of blood and tissues from all types of residual substances. All of this contributes then to treat arthritis, gallstones, arteriosclerosis, heart disease, cancer, and a variety of other ailments. If enzymes can treat and clean the body (removing toxins), they can more easily help us to avoid all these sufferings.

The younger an individual is, the more his body is rich in enzymes. As years pass and age increases, their numbers decrease progressively and, as they diminish, the power of life diminishes. Therefore, the elderly are those who especially need a diet rich in enzymes. Only in this way will they be protected from weariness and the typical discontent of old age.

The richest sources of enzymes are cereal sprouts, raw milk, egg yolk, vegetables, fruits, seeds, embryos, and mainly greens-based drinks.

A WORLD TO DISCOVER

For a better understanding of the world of enzymes, let us investigate deeper. In scientific terms, enzymes are protein molecules that are basically in charge of catalyzing all chemical reactions that occur within living organisms. Enzymes are capable of accelerating reactions that otherwise would require too much time or of reaching temperatures which are definitely not suitable for an individual to survive.

Their role consists in facilitating reactions through the interaction between the substrate (in biochemistry). Substrate defines a molecule on which an enzyme operates, and its active site—the part of the enzyme in which reactions take place—forms a complex.

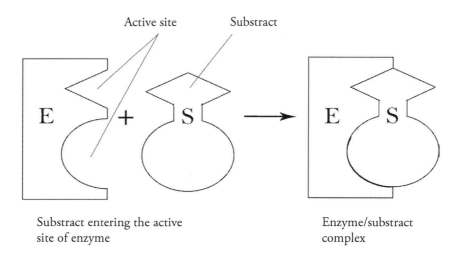

Substract entering the active   Enzyme/substract
site of enzyme   complex

Once the reaction takes place, the product is removed from the enzyme and the latter remains available to begin a new reaction. The simplest reaction catalyzed by an enzyme may be represented in this way:

$$E + S <====> ES <====> EP <====> E + P$$

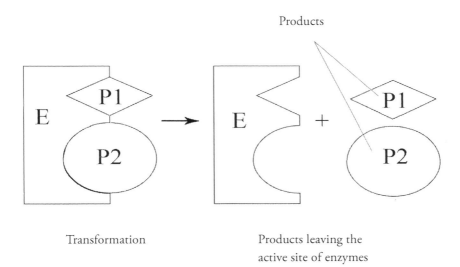

Transformation   Products leaving the
                  active site of enzymes

The enzyme is not consumed during the reaction. It combines the only reagent S and the substrate, in order to form an enzyme-substrate combination, ES. The ES is then transformed in EP, which then splits into the P product and into a free enzyme. The latter is again ready to react with another S molecule. The process takes place very quickly. In many cases, a single enzyme molecule can transform thousands of molecules of substrate into a product just in a second.

THE KEYS TO HEALTH

Enzyme activity can be compared to that of keys that open specific locks. Enzymes are long chains of proteins held together in specific forms by hydrogen bonds. If something happens to the hydrogen bonds, the enzymatic protein flakes, losing its shape.

Without a proper form, the key cannot open the lock. At that point, the enzyme cannot be distinguished anymore. It is just another foreign protein. At this moment, the body attacks itself because it perceives that there is a stowaway.

Enzymes have an important specificity. That is, each enzyme acts on a single substrate and during only one of the steps of a certain reaction. Therefore, for the regulation of metabolic pathways or of complex reactions, the coordinated activity of more types of enzymes is required. Not surprisingly, in each individual you can find over 2,000 different enzymes.

As we saw earlier, if bonds break, the enzyme falls apart and can no longer do its specific work. A broken-down enzyme is said to be denatured. There are various factors that denature an enzyme, for example, cooking foods at a temperature that exceeds 48 °C (118 °F). At a temperature of 45 °C (113 °F) enzymes become inactive.

Dr. Edward Howell, a known authority at a global level on enzymes and human nutrition, explains the process of denaturing of enzymes above 48 °C.[14]

Since water boils at 100 °C (212 °F), it is obvious that cooking damages all food, destroying the enzymes and the vitamins it contains. We already mentioned that only raw food can fully satisfy our organism with the necessary enzymes.

Therefore, the previous facts that are found to be true and which do not cause any economic benefit to science and industry are important to those of us who want to stay healthy.

There are many witnesses to healing through raw food. One

14 Howell, E., 1981. *Food Enzymes for Health and Longevity*. USA, Silver Lake, WI: Lotus Light Publications.

of these is the case in the U.S. of R. J. Cheatham who, at 40 years of age, was suffering from skin cancer. After several interventions in the outward part of the body, his scar came to measure almost 50 cm in length. Doctors didn't give him any chance to survive, so he found himself lying on his bed, waiting to die.

Cheatham tells how a book about fasting and treatment with the raw food diet ended up in his hands by chance. The book led him to read other similar books. After alternating fasting and consuming a diet of fresh juices and raw foods, Cheatham was healed.

Another important case is that of a Danish physician, Dr. Kristine Nolfi. In her book *My Experience with Living Food,*[15] the doctor wrote that she suffered from a breast cancer that had become as large as a hen's egg.

As a doctor, she was convinced that radiation and operations were only detrimental, and that their effect, at most, would only delay the progression of the disease. Hence, she chose to try the raw-food diet in order to be healed.

She writes, "At the expense of my own life, I had to demonstrate what a diet composed of 100 percent raw foods can achieve. During the first two months, the breast lump remained the same, and then the first signs of improvement appeared. The lump decreased and I regained my strength. My recovery was evident and I was feeling good, as I hadn't felt for many years."

After being totally healed, the doctor added to her natural diet 40 percent of cooked food. To her astonishment, the lump reappeared.

---

15 Nolfi, K., 2005. *My Experience with Living Food: Raw Food Treatment of Cancer.* USA, Pomeroy, WA: Health Research.

Therefore, she had to return at once to the rigid diet of raw foods. Eventually the tumor disappeared for the second time.

Thanks to this experience, Dr. Nolfi was convinced that raw food could cure any disease equally well. Subsequently, she opened a raw-food nursing home where all patients are still treated with 100 percent raw food and no medicines at all.

THE BEST BEAUTY TREATMENT

Through natural nutrition and fasting, any disease can be healed. Living food—raw food—is also the best beauty treatment: it accelerates cell renewal, the skin regains its elasticity, and wrinkle formation stops. Furthermore, glandular activity is balanced, eliminating the danger of obesity or excessive thinness. The more subtle and superficial blood vessels of the body, being better perfused, are polished by deposits. As a consequence we have a fresh and young appearance. Similarly, living food heals hypertension, angina pectoris, and can prevent myocardial infarction. Those who follow a natural diet of raw food experience a gradual rejuvenation that can lead to a reduction of biological age up to 20–30 years, even with regard to sexual activity.

In this chapter I introduced the functions of enzymes, a real miracle and a mystery before which man must recognize his own impotence. I also showed that taking exogenous enzymes, derived from foods and which help our body cells, is a law of nature. So it is up to each of us to decide whether or not the destruction of these enzymes through cooking, pasteurization, or other processes that we find in the food industry involves failure to comply with the laws of nature.

TO WHAT EXTENT ARE THE CHEMISTS RIGHT?

Due to the lack of enzymes in foods, the most important consequence is the loss of mineral salts, including phosphorus, calcium, potassium, iron, and so on, favoring in this way the generation of several diseases.

Chemists claim that cooking does not destroy the nutritive salts, and they are right. What is lost are the enzymes organically bound to salts. Without them, salts cannot be transformed and assimilated usefully, losing almost all their value and being deposited as residuals. Therefore, organic mineral nutritive salts are transformed into inorganic mineral ones.

Cooked foods, once metabolized, produce a large quantity of residues and acids that reach the blood. The elimination organs are not able to cope with such a big accumulation of residual substances. Therefore, the latter are deposited in great quantities in our body, causing various disturbances.

And what about doctors? The vast majority know nothing about the immense healing power of raw foods. Despite all the available knowledge and scientific experiments, most of the population has been left so far in total ignorance. On the other hand, it is also true that pathologies do not arise only because of the consumption of cooked foods.

Our body, as a normal consequence of its metabolism and partly as a natural defense against sickness, produces atoms and unstable molecules called *free radicals*. However, sometimes it overreacts, increasing their production and releasing a number of molecules and unstable atoms higher than necessary.

Some factors that can cause this overproduction are cigarette smoke, smog, diseases, and even intense physical activity. Free radicals contain at least one free electron, or negative charge, which makes them very reactive. As soon as they are produced, they seek other molecules with a positive charge with which to react, resulting in a reaction called oxidation. Free radicals can oxidize, or damage, the DNA and cell membranes, paving the way for cancer and other diseases.

It has been shown that free radicals are linked to aging, cancer, arteriosclerosis, hypertension, arthrosis, and immune deficiency. Enzymes and antioxidant compounds made of vitamins and organic minerals form the defense mechanisms against free radicals.

The importance of enzymes in cellular processes can be further demonstrated by the fact that the malfunctioning of a single enzyme, out of thousands, can cause a serious disease.

HALIME OLCAY

Halime Olcay was born on July 1, 1874, in eastern Turkey. In 2009 (latest available data) she was still alive.

It is impolite to ask the age of a lady; however, this does not apply to this lively grandma who in 2009 turned 135 years.

Her history was revealed by chance. The officials of the local Registry Office seeing no update of her identity document for 25 years and given her age to be included in the Guinness Book of Records, were convinced that the grandmother was dead by this time, so they stopped sending her the state pension. Halime Olcay went personally to complain. When she showed her documents, nobody in the office could believe that this independent old woman had twice the average lifespan of a Turkish person. Moreover, what vitality she had!

"I had to convince them that I was not dead yet. But they did not want to believe that I was so old," Halime said.

She speaks of her age more than willingly and with obvious pride. When she came into the world, the Sultan was still commanding the Ottoman Empire, and her people spoke Ottoman. We could say that in her life she saw all sorts of things, from the Independence War that led to the birth of modern Turkey, the two World Wars, the invasion of Cyprus, and the landing of the first man on the moon.

In an interview, Halime said that the thing she is most proud of is having seen closely, on two occasions, Mustafa Kemal Atatürk, the founder of modern Turkey, and even shaken hands with him.

"I remember it very well," she told the newspaper *Haber Turk*. "He was so handsome that when he arrived, we all touched him. And he was so kind. A true gentleman."

The mother of seven children, Halime lives with the last one who is still alive. He is 84 years old. Furthermore, she is surrounded by the affection of more than one hundred grandchildren and great-grandchildren. Despite her old age, she still has Prussian habits. She goes to bed early and gets up at dawn.

HER SECRET

During the interview,[16] while proudly waving her identity card that shows her date of birth, which seems to be almost a legend, the Turkish grandmother explained the reasons for her longevity: "I never go to the doctor because I do not trust doctors. I take care of myself with only natural remedies."

---

16 Yukuş, A., Akengin, İ., Nov 25, 2009. İşte dünyanın en yaşlı insanı. *Haber Turk*.

Then she added, "It all depends on what you eat. I consume just genuine foods that I produce by myself because I don't trust those that you normally buy. Every morning I have breakfast with raw milk and honey. Later I eat yogurt and vegetables from my garden. For dinner I like the bulgur pilaf, and I never eat after the prayer."

Halime's granddaughter affirms that her grandma's secret is also eating spinach, mushrooms, beets, and a lot of goat yogurt. She has always been in a good mood and has never lost her optimism.

DO PREGNANCY AGE WOMEN?

A careful reader will have noticed that both Sahan Dosova and Halime Olcay had many children. The first one had eleven children, whereas the second had seven.

But this is not all. In fact, the vast majority of women who have lived a long life have had several children.

Just to name a few more, the Brazilian Maria Olivia da Silva (130 years old) had ten children, the Canadian Marie-Louise Meilleur (117 years old) had ten, and the American Julia Huigens Tharnish (110 years old) had fourteen children.

There are many false beliefs that have to be debunked. In popular opinion one of these is the belief that the more children a woman has, the older she grows, and the weaker and uglier she becomes. The over-one-hundred-year-old ladies mentioned above show us the opposite. I don't mean that to get to an old age you have to bear ten children. Neither do I mean that to get there you have to avoid childbearing or have only a few children, as many may think.

On the contrary, I remember that the elderly ladies in our village, including my grandmother, used to recommend to sick women to get pregnant if they wanted to be healed. I was seven when I heard this advice for the first time. One day, in fact, I came back from school and I saw my grandmother talking to some elderly women. The oldest was about one hundred years old and the others were more or less the same age. Along with them there was a young woman about 40 years old.

"If you want to be healed, my dear, you have to get pregnant," said one of them to the young woman.

I realized from their conversation that this woman was very sick.

"Grandma, why should sick women get pregnant?" I asked.

The oldest of them turned towards me and said, "To renew the blood."

"What?" I asked, amazed.

"You see, pregnancy is like an elixir of youth. It cures diseases and reverses the clock of life," the old lady next to me answered.

I experienced a similar case firsthand in our family. My sister-in-law contracted hepatitis C in kindergarten when she was five years old. At that time, they still used to administer vaccines using only one syringe for an entire group of children. That time seven children were infected and one of them didn't survive.

Despite Natalia's health problems, my brother decided to

marry her. She always felt weak; sometimes she had to take medicines, and she was always pale. Moreover, she was often forced to stay in bed. When she got pregnant, my brother went to tell the news to our mother. He was worried about what he had been told by the doctors.

"You know, Natalia is pregnant. This is her third month."

"Congratulations! You are about to become a father," said our mother happily.

"But the doctor said that she must have an abortion immediately, otherwise she will die," he said sadly.[17]

"It's not true," replied my mother in anger.

"But her life is in serious danger."

"That is what doctors say! But I know many sick women who have been cured thanks to pregnancy. Many of them even seemed moribund and then we saw the miracles that happened. Your grandmother is right when she advises sick women to have a child." Our mother was convinced that this method would work also with her daughter-in-law.

From the very beginning my brother had encouraged Natalia to try our miraculous diet. She agreed even before she was married. Thanks to the new diet, her health improved significantly and she no longer had to take medicine.

Despite the doctors' advice, she decided to continue with her pregnancy. She was warned that the responsibility was entirely hers. My-sister-in-law lived every month of her pregnancy with the fear of dying and never seeing her son.

Instead, six months after the doctor's advice to abort the

---

17 The results of her medical exams were really worrying.

baby, Natalia gave birth to a wonderful baby boy. He was perfectly healthy and weighed 3.6 kg. The birth was natural. She did not have a C-section. In addition, the baby did not contract the Hepatitus C virus from his mother.

But the most interesting thing was that my sister-in-law felt much better than before her pregnancy. The doctors made her do all the necessary tests and even they were astonished that the results were all normal.

During pregnancy the virus was neutralized. It was still present, but it was as if it was "dead." The pregnancy had rejuvenated her.

After that successful experience, Natalia had two more children, another boy and a girl. She is still young, and if she wants she can have more children. Natalia was 18 years old when she had her first child and now she is 32.

With each childbirth, she felt better and better, and now she is completely healed. According to the exams, the virus "disappeared" entirely after the last birth.

Through this example we saw how through a combination of proper diet and pregnancy, many women may not only be healed from their diseases but also be rejuvenated by several years.

A recent study conducted by Israeli researchers of the Hadassah University Hospital revealed that women who give birth naturally after the age of 45 are likely to live longer than other women. It was highlighted that seven genes out of 60 in total showed significant differences between the women who gave birth after the age of 45 and those who had their last pregnancy when they were 30 years old. In particular, four of these genes would allow for inhibiting programmed cell death (apoptosis), allowing pregnancy after the age of 45, while the other three have a general longevity effect on woman.[18]

A few years ago, *Nature* published a study carried out in the U.S. with similar results. Women who had given birth between 40 and 45 years of age had a better chance of living a century. A similar study also came from China in 2004.[19]

In accordance with another study conducted by U.S. researchers of the Keck School of Medicine at the University of Southern California (USC),[20] women who gave birth between 30 and 40 years of age and, if possible, even beyond that age, decreased the risk of endometrial cancer from 17 percent to 44 percent over women who had their last child before the age of 25. Risk reduction seems to be age-dependent. That is, the older the age at which a woman gives birth to her last child, the lower the risk.

In particular, researchers found that after the age of 30 years, the risk of endometrial cancer begins to decrease by about thirteen percentage points for every five years of late births. Regarding women who give birth before the age of 25, those who have their last child

---

18 Even, D., April 10, 2012. *Israeli Researchers Discover Anti-Aging Genes in Ultra-Orthodox Women*, "Haaretz."

19 Yi, Z., Vaupellyac, J. W., 2004. "Association of late childbearing with healthy longevity among the oldest-old in China," *Population Studies: A Journal of Demography*, Vol. 58, Issue 1, pp. 37-53. Taylor & Francis Group.

20 Wendy Setiawan, V. W., et al., 2012. "Age at Last Birth in Relation to Risk of Endometrial Cancer: Pooled Analysis in the Epidemiology of Endometrial Cancer Consortium," *American Journal of Epidemiology* [online]. Internet website: http://aje.oxfordjournals.org/content/early/2012/07/23/aje.kws129

between the ages of 30 and 34 years have a probability of risk reduction of 17 percent, while those who give birth between 35 and 39 years of age instead have a probability of risk reduction of 32 percent.

"We found that the lowest risk of endometrial cancer persisted even for the oldest mothers among the different age groups including those under 50, 50–59, 60–69, and over 70 years of age, which shows that protection persists for many years," declares the USC public announcement by Dr. Wendy Setiawan, leading researcher of the study.

In another study, T. Perls and his colleagues showed that women who have lived 100 years or more, gave birth four times more often after the age of 40 than those who did not live more than 73 years.

The relationship between giving birth and the life span of a woman can be explained easily. By nature, the most important thing is that the organism can procreate, and then it can also leave the scene. So it seems that nature has developed mechanisms to prevent ageing, at least until the woman gives birth. But the condition is that the women follow a proper diet, like the one explained in our book.

After the age of 40, it is more likely that a woman is "blocked" from residues and toxins, that her DNA is damaged and contains errors. Despite the fact that the woman would only benefit from giving birth, the child may be born with malformations.

Frolkis, a famous Russian gerontologist, has said: "We know that the higher the mother's age at conception, the greater the risk of genetic abnormalities in her offspring. Therefore, the genetic risk, depending on the age of the mother, increases from 0.1 percent in women who are below 35 years old to 3.5 percent in those aged 45 (35 times higher)."

Consequently, women who follow a wrong diet and decide to have children after they are 40 years old are likely to give birth to children affected with Down syndrome and other malformations. That is why it is advisable to follow the diet we propose in this text for at least one year before becoming pregnant.

Before the era of food additives and other junk food, all that we have said above was not necessary! DNA errors appeared with civilization. It is interesting to note that in Eastern Europe, where the food industry is less sophisticated as compared to the West, mothers give birth to healthy children until menopause. In these countries, Down syndrome is almost unknown.

The only problem with having many children is the unsustainable growth of the world population, but that is beyond the scope of interest of this book.

CHAPTER 3

ACIDS IN THE HUMAN ORGANISM

All deaths are due to a situation of progressive organic acidity.
Dr. W. Crile

To assimilate and use nutrients, our body needs to transform food into an acidic or alkaline solution, depending on the type of food ingested.

We can determine if a food is acid or alkaline by examining the residual ashes after its digestion. What does this mean? It means that all food, once "burned" into the human organism, leaves a residue, defined as ashes, which can be neutral, acidic, or alkaline, depending on the mineral composition of the food. If the ashes prevail over alkaline minerals—sodium, potassium, calcium, and magnesium—they are alkaline. If they prevail over mineral acids—sulfur, phosphorus, chlorine, organic acids not metabolized—they are considered acidic.

In order to maintain the acid/base equilibrium of the body—80 percent basic and 20 percent acid—at least 80 percent of the food we consume should produce alkaline ashes. Why?

Our bodies have been created alkaline. It is true that we also generate acid through the gastric glands, but this is only to help with digestion. Thus, apart from the stomach, no other part of the body should be acidic.

ACID/BASE EQUILIBRIUM OF THE HUMAN BODY

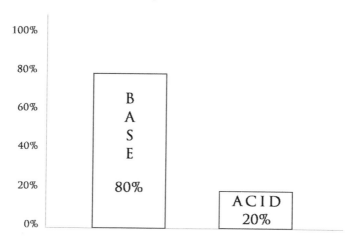

This is why a person should always have high reserves of alkaline substances and limit foods that produce acids.

The most widespread and insidious factor that contributes to the emergence of various diseases of our society is *acidosis*, which consists of a stockpile of acid that the body cannot assimilate effectively.

A REAL PLAGUE FOR HUMANITY

Medicine generally considers acidosis as a pathological condition. Many people think that it is a normal condition, but they are wrong.

Actually, this condition anticipates almost all chronic degenerative diseases, including cancer, diabetes, arthritis, and heart disease. These pathologies are so widespread as to be considered a real plague for humanity.

Acidosis is not often evident because the patient feels well in the early stages of acid accumulation. In fact, he can feel excessively well and still have an unusually high level of energy.

Unfortunately, this is a wrong perception resulting from the "stimulating" reaction of the body control system that works very quickly to remove the excess of acid. Both the well-being state and the outstanding energy disappear when additional acid keeps accumulating.

Because of the ongoing effort to maintain the necessary alkalinity, the neutralizing alkaline reserves become exhausted and the liver becomes congested and loses its ability to carry out its detoxification function. When the intracellular and extracellular fluids lose their alkalinity, a person is considered to be in a condition of acidosis.

THE CONSEQUENCES

The human body cannot allow that its acid/basic equilibrium be disturbed. Therefore, it has to act as soon as possible to neutralize the excess of acids. This neutralization is performed by mobilizing some alkaline substances and various mineral salts from the body reserves.

For example, alkalizing minerals such as calcium, potassium, sodium, and magnesium are subtracted from the bones, teeth, and the cells of all tissues. Even the excretory organs—kidneys, skin, intestine, etc.—are subject to overwork in an attempt to eliminate the excess of dangerous acids and minerals due to the neutralization processes.

The mucous membranes of these organs, to which we should add the bronchial tube, the salivary and lacrimal glands, the uterus, and so on, are clearly damaged by corrosive substances which lead to the ideal conditions for a variety of ailments such as skin problems, the so-called microbial infections, inflammation, gallstones, or kidney stones.

ACIDS OPEN THE DOOR TO CANCER

Our bodies are composed of seventy-five trillion cells held together by connective tissue. When the defense system and the cleaning are overloaded or too slow, the connective tissue becomes a real theater of inflammatory and degenerative pathologies. Furthermore, nutritional exchanges are altered so that cells are poorly nourished and oxygenated and are immersed in an intoxicated environment.

Dr. Otto Warburg, winner of the Nobel Prize in medicine, declared[21] that cancer arises from the incapacity of the cell to breathe, that is, to receive osmotically the extracellular fluid that causes lack of oxygen to the cell.

Two factors are always present in cancer: an acidic pH (potential of hydrogen) and lack of oxygen. Cancer needs an acid environment with little oxygen in order to survive and grow.

Patients with terminal cancer are about a thousand times more acidic when compared to healthy people. As a matter of fact,

---

21 Warburg, O., 10 Dec 1931. *The Oxygen-transferring Ferment of Respiration.* Lecture at Nobel Prize Award; June 30, 1966. *The Prime Cause and Prevention of Cancer.* Lecture to Nobel Laureates. Lindau, Germany.

the majority of patients suffering from cancer present a very low physiological pH. Why is it so?

In the absence of oxygen, glucose is submitted to fermentation in lactic acid. This causes the pH of the cell to fall from 7.3 to 7.2 to 7 and then to 6.5 in the later stages of the disease. In the case of metastasis, the pH drops to 6.0 and even to 5.7 or less.

Our bodies simply cannot fight the disease if the pH is not properly balanced. A healthy human cell has lots of molecular oxygen and a pH which is slightly alkaline. A cancerous cell has an acid pH and lack of oxygen.

Cancer cells cannot survive in an environment rich in oxygen. Increasing the pH and the oxygen concentration from 7.4 upward, we can create a hostile environment for cancer which, instead, would thrive in anaerobic conditions characterized by of lack of oxygen, namely, acidic conditions. Mushrooms, precursors of cancer, thrive in an acid environment.

THERE IS NO NATURAL DEATH

It has now been accepted by many authorities that diseases are developed because of a reduction of the organic functions and of a lowering of the body resistance as a result of a condition of chronic acidosis. In this regard, Dr. George W. Crile, head of the Crile Clinic in Cleveland and one of the most famous surgeons in the world, declared that, "There is no natural death. All death cases defined in that way are only the ending point of a progressive acidification of the organism."[22]

---

22 This famous statement is cited in many books about health.

When the level of toxins in our bodies reaches the tolerable maximum, the body starts a cleaning action that may take several forms. For example, these can be diarrhea, headache, colds, skin eruptions, abscesses, boils, rheumatism, inflammation of the eyes or of other organs, colds, chills, fever, and all the complex series of symptoms that are recognized by the names of the various diseases. All these problems, however, have a common origin: accumulation of acidic waste in the organism.

Uric acid represents the largest part of the excess of acids. To this are added other substances foreign to the body, such as salt, various toxins, and poisons.

Excessive and unbalanced eating, together with excessive nervous stress, are the conditions for a large intoxication that in turn generates inflammatory processes that are nothing but attempts to purify the body. When an anti-inflammatory drug stops the process, or when the load of toxins is really excessive, toxins accumulate and migrate to deeper tissues and can lead to degenerative diseases.

All acids are deposited "illegally" throughout the body forming residues, "caps" of mucus, calcifying tissues, covering the walls of the arteries or other organs with fats; some acids are deposited in joints and muscles in crystal form. Thus the entire normal physiological activity of every organ is overloaded. It is no wonder that joint pain comes about, that atherosclerosis arises, that kidneys no longer function properly, that injuries do not heal, that kidney stones and gallstones appear, that lumps are formed, and that fatigue and headaches become uninvited and permanent guests.

Chemical and pharmaceutical products are of little help and, in general, they favor the emergence of other diseases. Even in this case, true healing is achieved only by eliminating the cause of the disease. Then nature will work in favor of our health.

EAT AND YOU WILL FEEL BETTER

Today food has become more a fashion than a necessity. We often eat just for the pure pleasure that such action procures to the palate. Therefore, many do not care if some foods are healthy or not.

The overwhelming majority of the foods an average individual consumes is mostly of industrial origin. It is rich in acids, preservatives, dyes, and lots of other rubbish. Eating these unhealthy and refined foods is equal to opening the door of our health to all kinds of diseases in the world. The frantic pace of life today is not only due to stress, but it is also due to bad eating habits.

With each passing day, the food and beverages we consume are becoming more "acid producers," especially quick meals such as those offered by fast food restaurants and precooked foods. Sweets and desserts create acid too, as well as coffee, wine, and beer.

Another element that creates acidity is overeating, i.e., eating more solid foods which lack liquids than necessary. Note that even those who follow a vegetarian diet can end up with a high level of acidity if they consume too much grain.

Worries, anxiety, fear, and intense and/or chronic stress are other factors that can produce organic acidity, and so are the pollutants and any toxins in the environment where we live.

TELL ME WHAT YOU EAT AND I WILL TELL YOU WHAT CHARACTER YOU HAVE

It has also been demonstrated that a prolonged period of acidosis not only affects the physical condition but also the mental and emotional state of the patient. And, conversely, the attitude can affect the physical condition. This means that a person can follow a diet rich in fruits and vegetables but still remain in an acid diet. Regardless of the type of the diet used; the person who has a negative view of life turns out to be acidic.

Negative thoughts, in fact, stimulate the action of the adrenal glands, which in turn accelerate the metabolic activity of our body. When this happens, more acid is produced. And, since the process is continuous, the amount of acid increases.

It can be a vicious circle, a perpetual one: the more acidic we become, the more negative we are. And the more negative, defensive, argumentative, and unpleasant we are, the more acidic we will become. A pessimistic person who looks at everything with negativity is almost certainly in a state of acidosis.

Consequently, ingested food affects not only physical condition, but the brain and mind as well. Namely, it affects our personality and behavior because it can favor a good mood or arouse enthusiasm, have a calming effect and/or reduce inflammation, or it can cause irritation and be a contributing cause of inflammation.

For example, meat causes aggressiveness and inflames the intestinal mucosa due to the putrefaction that it induces. On one hand, it gives an apparent force, as a whip or a drug. But on the other hand, it induces aggressiveness, like the excitation of the villi and of the neurons of the enteric nervous system present in the intestine.

Sausages, especially pork, cause nervousness, irritability, aggressiveness, and insomnia, not to mention the processes of putrefaction, inflammation, and irritation that they cause in the intestine. If we eat meat we will be more aggressive and led to a predatory sexuality, whereas eating vegetables and carbohydrates leads to a more playful sexuality.

This has been demonstrated in a high school that is well-known as "problematic" in the United States. There the canteen started a reevaluation program of the school: only biological foods, very little meat, and no complex sugars were offered. After a short time, the aggressiveness of the students was drastically reduced. This means that blood and meat make us fierce.

THE THERMOMETER OF HEALTH

We can control our acid/basic equilibrium by testing the scale of measure of the pH which was created in 1909 by the famous Danish chemist Søren Sørensen. The pH usually takes values between 0 (strong acid) and 14 (strong base). The condition of neutrality corresponds to the intermediate value of approximately 7.0. In human beings, for example, the pH of the blood must remain constant at a value of 7.4; otherwise one may die.

It is worth recalling that old age is also the result of the chronic loss of bicarbonate in the blood and of the continuous rise of acidosis together with intoxication that produces inflammation.

The best way to control the acidity of our bodies is to control the acidity in the urine, a test that can be done easily by anyone.

Follow the advice of my books and you will no longer need to do any analysis, checkups, or tests because all your values will be automatically normal.

We can measure the pH of our urine with an electronic pH meter (*pH-meter*) or with simple litmus paper that can be purchased at the pharmacy, although the first method is more convenient and practical. We have to analyze the second urine of the morning and at least two more times a day, once before lunch and again before dinner. Then we calculate the average of our readings. We have to repeat this measurement for 10–15 days because acidosis is highly variable and depends on what we ate the night before.

If we use litmus paper instead, simply detach a piece of strip from the roll and wet its tip while urinating. The wet part changes color. There is a color chart printed on the packaging where we can detect and mark the corresponding number on the card that we will prepare. For the health of our bodies it is essential that the pH of our urine does not fall below 7.

There are numerous causes of acidification,
a) The consumption of acidifying foods (animal protein, sugar, tea, coffee, alcohol).
b) The lack of trace elements and vitamins.
c) Chelating substances originated from pollution.
d) Lack of oxygenation in inactive persons.
e) Endocrine insufficiency.
f) Excessive physical fatigue.
g) Disorders of the excretory organs (e.g., renal failure).
h) Use of chemical drugs.
i) Several psychological conditions (anger, worry, fear, etc.).

CONSEQUENCES OF AN ACID PH

An acid pH:
1. Corrodes arteries, veins, and heart tissue.
2. Accelerates the damage of free radicals.
3. Accelerates premature aging.
4. Causes weight gain, diabetes, and obesity.
5. Affects blood pressure.
6. Causes the formation of cholesterol plaques.
7. Inhibits the metabolism of stored energy reserves.
8. Inhibits cell regeneration and the synthesis of DNA-RNA.
9. Inhibits the activity of vital electrolytes.
10. Prevents oxygen from reaching the tissues.
11. Modifies the metabolism of lipids and fatty acids.
12. Causes all forms of cancer.
13. Causes senility, dementia, and Alzheimer's disease.
14. Causes osteoporosis, osteoarthritis, and tooth loss.
15. Numerous other ailments.

According to Dr. G. Enderlein's research,[23] total healing of chronic diseases occurs only when the blood is returned to a normal pH, which is slightly alkaline.

23 Enderlein, G., 1955–1959. *Akmon*, Volume I–III. Germany, Hamburg: Ibica-Verlag.

A PERFECT BALANCE

Among all foods, raw milk is the only one that, once metabolized, has an acid-base ratio corresponding exactly to that of the blood. That's because milk is the only type of food for infants for a long period of time.

After the process of metabolization, from certain foods we obtain only acid substances, from others only base ones, and from many others we get both categories of substances. Therefore, it is important to know exactly what we get from each food so that we can choose our diet carefully.

In accordance with some research, there are tables containing the acid-base ratio of foods. With the help of these tables we can classify foods in the following way,

Foods that give 100 percent acid substances:

Meat

Animal fat

Vegetable fat

White bread

Panettone

Refined sugar

Soft drinks

Coffee

Cocoa

Tea

Wine

Alcoholic drinks

Table salt
Bitter fruits
Desserts prepared with sugar
Chocolate

Foods that are transformed 100% to bases:

All types of greens and vegetables
Onions
Potatoes
Chestnuts
Bran cereals
Seed sprout (except the pods of legumes)

The composition of all other types of foods swings between acidic and basic components, whereas milk, because it corresponds to the percentage existing in the blood, is considered neutral.

These foods are considered almost neutral:

Ripe bananas
Melons
Cucumbers
Tomatoes
Very ripe apples (not green ones)

Patients must be very careful when they choose their food. Cereal gives 60 percent of base substances, although with cooking the basic value decreases considerably. But we must not be slaves of the acid-base ratio of food tables. Hippocrates didn't know anything about calories or the acid/base ratio of the food, yet he knew perfectly how to cure a diabetic.

If, exceptionally, we are offered foods belonging to the first group (acids), we can, of course, eat them, but with moderation because otherwise our bodies cannot cope with the excess of acids and might fail to neutralize or eliminate the acids.

One of the most serious consequences of hyperacidity is the loss of calcium, which, as a consequence, is subtracted from the bones and teeth in order to neutralize the excess of acids. Other pathologies that emerge are, for example: nerve diseases, tooth diseases, spinal column pain, fractures occurring easily, and many others.

For patients who want to recover, it is better if they do not touch any of the foods in question. To those affected by rheumatism, arthritis, bone and dental diseases, I advise following a diet based on basic food as much as possible. People who really want to be healed have to renounce everything that is cooked.

It seems that the majority of people find it is impossible to change their diet, switching to a regime of only raw vegetables. In fact, it seems that they prefer the pain, injections, and suffering.

At most, when they approach death and pain becomes unbearable, and doctors and medicines can no longer help them, people are overwhelmed by despair and begin to be interested in this diet. Many of them, however, could be saved and they could help themselves by following the above advice.

SHIRALI MUSLIMOV

Shirali Muslimov (March 26, 1805–September 2, 1973), was a Talysh shepherd (native of the Caucasus from Iranian ethnicity) from the Republic of Azerbaijan. Yes, Shirali Muslimov lived 168 years. The extra-super-centenarian was born and raised in Barzavu, a small village in the region of Lerik in a mountainous area of Azerbaijan, near the Iranian border. According to him, his parents lived for a long time as well. His father lived more than 110 years and his mother more than 90 years.

Born in 1805, during the time of Tsar Alexander I, he outlived five Russian tzars, Lenin, and Stalin. Shirali became ill with pneumonia during the winter of 1972–1973. However, he survived at least until his 168th birthday, dying in late summer. Since he was 18 years old he was a quiet shepherd of his sheep on the slopes and mountains of the Caucasus every day, walking along with his herd about 10–15 kilometers.

The Muslimov case became known in 1963 when a young photo reporter for TASS, Kelman Kaspiev, went to Barzavu to interview the elderly. There were old certificates attesting the incredible fact that a man born in 1805 was still alive at the age of 158 years. The Soviet government was not the only one interested in his history. Even *National Geographic* showed a big interest toward it, although later it stepped off, mainly for political reasons rather than other causes, as the Soviets began to make this "Methuselah" a propaganda tool for the regime. Nevertheless, the grandfather apparently was not a big supporter of the Soviet system. In fact, Kaspiev asked him during the interview, "When were you better, then or now?"

"In the past I had 100–150 sheep," said the old man, "but one day a man came to me riding a horse [the Soviet regime] and took from me half of the herd. Now things are better, because no one can take anything away from me anymore."

Kaspiev's report, however, changed the life of the small village in Azerbaijan because finally electricity, radio, and television reached the village. Furthermore, a wide road was built, which would be of use to many curious people and for the same government institutions that wanted to meet and honor the man they thought was the most long-lived person in the world.

The old man was given many gifts and a special pension. In 1964, the Soviet government organized a big party for his 159th birthday. The small village of Barzavu soon became a tourist attraction, but also a gerontological mecca.

For decades, Soviet scientists and others from the West stopped in Barzavu to converse with the tireless Muslimov, gathering information about his diet, lifestyle, and sexual habits.

During his lifetime, Shirali had three wives and more than 200 family members: children, grandchildren, great-grandchildren and great-great-grandchildren. The last time he got married he was 136 years old, whereas his wife, Hatum Nuryeva, was 57 years old. From her he had a daughter during the first year of marriage. His wife lived to be 104 years and she was seven years older than one of this man´s grandchildren.

Regardless of the unlikelihood of this case, the Guinness Book of Records does not consider any of this evidence truthful since no Western scientist was able to examine the old man closely. In my opinion, the true reason was the fear of the Soviets that people from the West could find before them the secret formula of longevity. We all know that during the Cold War there was fierce competition between the Soviet Bloc and the West.

However, after the death of Shirali Muslimov the province of Lerik left to the gerontologists another thousand super-centenarians to study. Other people who have lived a long life in the same region are: Mahmud Eivasov, 152 years; Majid Agayeva, 144 years; and Nanii Ahmedova, 120 years. All of them were born in the favorable province of Lerik and passed away after having lived a long life.

This is why in Lerik a museum of super-centenarians was opened. It has no equal in the world. The main exhibits of the museum are letters, telegrams, books, essays, newspapers, and photographs that tell the life of the elderly people who lived in the town.

HIS SECRET

In January 1973, the venerable Shirali Muslimov was examined by a group of doctors. The doctors were shocked that the organism of the 168-year-old mountaineer functioned as the body of a teenager! Shirali Muslimov gladly shared with them the secret of his unprecedented longevity: "We must always work; idleness generates laziness and laziness produces death."

In fact, this extraordinary man worked tirelessly in the vicinity of his village until his last days. In that village, surrounded by the Talysh Mountains, the shepherd lived 168 years eating only raw and genuine food, such as milk, cheese, yogurt, fruits, and vegetables.

Instead of sugar he ate only honey and did not use salt; he drank only fresh spring water and infusions of marinated herbs. He did not smoke and, as a good Muslim, he did not drink alcohol. He bathed in spring water and slept under the open sky. He maintained a philosophical attitude toward life that helped him avoid all unnecessary worry and stress.

In Soviet times, a documentary about him was filmed, entitled *Shirali Comes Down from the Mountains* (*Ширали спускается с гор*).

DO PEOPLE WHO WORK LIVE LONGER THAN OTHERS?

Many people think that the more we work, the more our bodies will be consumed. But if we look at what people over a hundred years old do and say about work, we find that exactly the opposite is true. From his experience Shirali Muslimov said, "We must always work; idleness generates laziness and laziness generates death."

It seems to us that we age quickly because we do work a lot, but this is another "deaf fly" case. The truth is that when we do not work we age faster. Sitting in an office for eight hours, five days a week, and then spending the remaining two days glued in front of the TV or the computer at home hurts us.

People who have a sedentary lifestyle, like the one we mentioned, are usually weak and get sick more often. For this reason, in the late 1970s corporate gyms appeared in the United States. Today, many far-sighted managers arrange for a gym at their company for their employees.

As early as 2001 in the United States, more than 81 percent of companies with at least 50 employees had adopted programs to improve the health of their workers—a choice dictated by the potential benefits for both the employee and the company.

Stress management, better cardiovascular conditions, joint flexibility, and weight control are, in fact, some of the advantages for the physical wellness of employees who practice fitness at the office.

Gyms are luminous and pleasant places. Furthermore, going there is also a great way to improve relationships with colleagues. Employees are more relaxed and friendly, which eventually is useful in terms of productivity.

The ability to carry out physical activity at the gym of the company also reduces the number of mistakes made while working and cheers people up. All this means lots of advantages for the company, most of all in the reduction of healthcare costs and absenteeism due to illness.

A study on longevity led by Duke University shows that the first factor—chosen among a list of 788 different factors—associated with an especially long life is satisfaction in the work we do. Job satisfaction, therefore, is ranked in first place, prevailing over factors such as good health habits and genetics.

Choosing public transport to get to work will help to keep a person healthier. This is not the usual environmental or health warning; it is the result of a study conducted by a group of Canadian researchers and published in the *Journal of Public Health Policy*.[24] Walking to the bus stop or subway brings significant benefits, either environmental or concerning health. It is estimated that, in general, those who travel by public transport have to walk at least 30 minutes.

It is the 30 minutes of daily physical activity that is necessary to avoid the danger of a sedentary lifestyle. Of course, a person needs to walk at a rapid pace. According to the experts at the University of California, Berkeley, walking at a rate of one-kilometer-and-a-half every quarter of an hour (i.e., about six and a half kilometers per hour) will burn about the same number of calories as does jogging.

In this way, we can avoid gym registration fees and the costs related to the daily use of the car and we can also decrease pollution. So both our health and our economy make a profit out of this. People who have the opportunity can commute to work on foot or on a bicycle.

I use a bike to go to work and pedal 16 km per day, from Monday to Saturday. My wife bikes 25 km per day and some friends of mine do even more than 40 km a day. We usually use the car only for shopping or when we leave town.

The benefits we can get from moderate physical activity such as walking or riding a bike include the reduction of cholesterol levels and body weight, the stimulation of the immune system, bone strengthening, and improvement of our sense of humor. We can notice the first benefits in mood change. By moving, walking, or swimming we release endorphins, i.e., hormones that help us control stress and

24 Lachapelle U., Frank L. D., 2009. "Transit and Health: Mode of Transport, Employer-Sponsored Public Transit Pass Programs, and Physical Activity," *Journal of Public Health Policy*, 30, S73-S94.

anxiety, improving the overall feeling of well-being.

Another study was also published that examined the benefits in terms of life extension that can be attributed to an active lifestyle. In this case, the survey was conducted among the population of the famous Framingham study group. The selected persons were at least 50 years old, with different risk factors known and affected by other diseases from cancer to hypertrophy of the left ventricle.

Regardless of other risk factors and comorbidities, people doing moderate activity gained 1.3 years of life, while those doing more exercise gained 3.7 years in the case of men and 3.5 years in the case of women, compared to sedentary people.

It is true that work is tiring, but it is equally true that it extends life. The above statement has been scientifically proven. According to some researchers from three international American and German universities, who analyzed many data, in countries with greater or full employment, both average life and life expectancy are higher. Even in cases of increased productivity, life is longer. On the contrary, in countries that are struggling with pandemic or creeping unemployment, life expectancy decreases.

Someone might argue that countries in which there is a lot of work are wealthier and have better living conditions. However, the direct correlation between life and work is unmistakable. People who work, and especially if they work hard, live longer.

Work is the activity that keeps the brain alive, together with its mental and physical faculties. Certainly it is a matter of measurement. A person forced to work 15 hours a day in unacceptable personal and environmental conditions runs the risk of not making it or suffering disabilities.

DO PEOPLE WHO WORK LIVE LONGER?

In accordance with the German scientist James Vaupel, someone who works longer and retires as late as possible can surely hope for a long life, much longer than the life of the "baby" pensioner. So work, and above all hard work, is good for our health and for our wallet. Vaupel´s studies have confirmed that, thanks to work, life expectancy is longer.

In conclusion, work, work, work, according to the German style. And when a person eventually retires, what will he do? Vaupel answers that we should immediately cultivate new interests and alternative activities to replace the job we left. The human being is like a machine. The important thing is that it should never stop. The benefit we get can be expressed in money but, above all, in good health.

CHAPTER 4

HUMAN NUTRITION

The time will come when man will no longer have to kill
in order to eat, and even the killing of one animal will be
considered a major crime.

Leonardo da Vinci

Then God said, "Behold, I have given you every herb bearing seed,
which is upon the face of the earth and every tree, in which is the fruit
of the tree yielding seed: shall it be your food." This was the first lesson
on nutrition that our Creator gave the first couple of human beings,
cited as it is written on the first page of the Bible (see Genesis 1:29).

Herbs and fruits, together with cereals, should be man's food,
but they do not have to be treated or cooked. Rather, they should
be left as they naturally are. This teaching of the Bible represents the
key that opens the door to well-being and longevity. The verse shows
us that God, who created us and knows how we are made, tells us
what to eat and what not to eat. We can make a comparison with
the inventor of the gasoline engine. The engineer knows better than

anyone else how the engine is made and how it works. For this reason, he tells us to use gasoline and not alcohol or Coca-Cola; otherwise, the engine will break down.

TRUE OR FALSE?

Can human life really reach 120 years? Yes, it can. It has been demonstrated either by the scientific point of view, thanks to the experiments conducted on various animals, or from the practical point of view, confirmed by the super-centenarians of our days.

But the story does not end there. In the Bible we find the confirmation of such things. The Lord said, "My spirit shall not contend with man forever, for he is flesh; his days shall be a hundred and twenty years"[25] (see Genesis 6:3).

Since there was a time when people used to eat more meat obtained from hunting (baked or fried meat), it could be said that man's nutrition based on meat and its cooking was a normal thing. Similar conclusions have little foundation and, therefore, are even more perplexing.

Why do wild animals, which live in freedom, not usually get sick, while among the civilized nations of today we can hardly find an individual who is still healthy? To get the correct answer to this question it can be useful to make some comparisons with what happens in the animal world.

Which category of animals is more akin to man with regard to the anatomy and physiology of the digestive system? Is it, maybe, the category of predators, herbivores, omnivores (e.g., pork), or those that are nourished mainly by fruits (e.g., monkeys)?

25 We can find cases of extreme longevity in all the religions of the world.

Gorillas, for example, never eat meat. In addition, the anthropoid monkey is the only animal whose digestive system is made and works exactly like man's system.

The intestine of carnivores is five times shorter than that of humans; their molars are jagged, while man's are rounded. Their saliva is acidic, and man's is alkaline. Their intestine is smooth on the inside, while man's is pleated. Their tongue is rough to touch, whereas man's is sharp and smooth. In addition, the gastric acid is more acidic, i.e., it is stronger in predators.

Since the hydrochloric acid is too weak in man for the digestion of meat, and his intestine is pleated and five times longer than that of carnivorous animals, meat remains too long in our intestines, producing rot and a bad smell. The rotten substances then pass into the blood through the intestinal wall, causing various diseases.

Herbivorous animals do not have nails to catch and tear to pieces their prey. Man and monkeys are the only animals with hands that can climb on trees to take fruits. This proves that in their diet they first of all need fruit.

Civilization has brought about fundamental changes in man's lifestyle; however, the shape of their digestive tract has remained the same. So far it is equal to that of anthropoid monkeys. As a consequence, man's diet should be composed of fruits and vegetables. Among these we should include nuts and seeds as well.

The monkey feeds on seeds, roots, and leaves too, which would correspond to our salad. It has nothing to do with cooking, table salt, refined sugar, or preservatives.

With regard to humans, we can say that we can be much

healthier the less our food has gone through preparation processes. These words have the value of the laws of nature because we are created to consume the same type of food. This applies to the entire world living on Earth. No animal species can live a long time if they eat cooked foods, stored and processed ones, and so on.

A LEAP INTO THE PAST

All the theories and the hypotheses on nutrition of prehistoric man that large economic forces, and a science submitted to power and profits, have tried to force us to accept are false. We should start with an undeniable fact: our ancient ancestors were not carnivores, neither were they herbivores nor omnivores. They were simply frugivorous, and they were like that for many years, the first of their existence.

They lived in the forest, which gave them the food to which the human species is biologically adapted, namely, the juicy and sweet fruit that still today we instinctively seek and have sought since we were children, as long as we keep our healthy food instincts.

Therefore, we are still born frugivorous. Since we were children we have wanted and preferred fruit instead of meat because we are attracted uniquely to the food that best suits our physio-mental structure and thus is nutritionally optimal.

No doubt, for each animal species there is a suitable food, one which suits better than any other. From the scientific point of view, this is easily explained since there is a strict, deep, and atavistic correlation between a certain type of food and the anatomically functional structure of the animal that eats it. This relationship constitutes a guarantee of conservation and health to the organism in question that, therefore, is obviously attracted instinctively to that specific food.

That organism is prepared, according to a natural law and in an optimal way, to the ingestion and digestion of that specific food on top of any other. Prehistoric man used to eat mostly fruits but also vegetables and seeds. His diet varied according to the season, essentially based on the availability of food.

WHY HAS MAN BECOME CARNIVOROUS?

In the long period during which man fed only on fruit in his native habitat, the inter-tropical fruitful forest, only the protein content of fruits, vegetables, and seeds covered his protein requirement.

Let us try to understand the reasons for the advent of carnivorous eating in human life, a thing that has all the characteristics of a tragic decline and from which the physio-psychic degeneration of man started.

During human prehistory, meteorological and geological events occurred that profoundly altered the environment. Especially, vegetal biomes were altered. From them, man used to take his nourishment.

What took place was:

- Glaciations (glacial expansions)
- Interglacial periods (glacial retreat and the advent of warmer climates)
- Periods of strong drying climate (drought)
- Periods of exceptional rise of rainfall

For man, the last glaciation was particularly important. That huge glaciation caused the advancing of the glaciers over a great part of the Eurasian regions. It brought about the destruction of forests, effects which lasted until 10,000 years ago.

Contemporaneous to that glaciation were the very intense precipitation (rainfall) that took place in Africa, and these weather events had many consequences for man. A dramatic scarcity of rain and the subsequent drying of the climate followed the rainfall. All of these events resulted in large reductions of forests, which turned mostly into savannahs.

In order to survive, man was forced to act like an animal living in the savannah, feeding himself on what was available in that environment. There he found grasses, plants that require open space and direct sunlight, conditions offered by the savannah and certainly not offered by the shadow forest from where man came.

Grasses produce dried fruits, odorless and tasteless. They are, hence, food for birds. With various tricks man could also, with the aid of fire, use the grains. However, the most revolutionary event that occurred to man, because he behaved like an animal of the savannah, was turning to meat as his food. Man became, out of necessity, a meat eater. But always with the aid of fire because he was not able to eat either raw grains or meat.

Without the help of cooking and milling for cereal, man would not have become either a meat eater or a cereal eater, because his natural anatomical features (teeth, etc.) alone would not have allowed this transformation.

THE COST OF SURVIVAL

The impact of the unnatural deviations of food—grains and proteins of animal carcasses, moreover cooked, i.e., dead food—had catastrophic consequences for humans in terms of health and lifespan. This is understandable, given the overhanging leap from live and vitalizing foods to those starchy and meaty, cadaveric and deadly foods high in protein, such as meat, killed and then devitalized with cooking.

Reay Tannahill in his *Food in History*[26] tells us, "During the period of the Neanderthals, less than half of the population over the age of 20 survived, and nine out of ten of the remaining adults died before the age of 40."

It was mainly the advent of meat with its excessive content of proteins and the resulting toxemia that produced such disastrous effects not only on the human body but also on the minds of men. We must not, in fact, forget that meat leads to aggressiveness.

As the influential anthropologist James Collier said, "As a consequence of the disastrous effects of these upsetting events on climate and vegetation, man could no longer rely on plants to live and had to resort to meat."

However, man is powerless. He is not carnivorous by nature because anatomically he lacks the suitable equipment to chase, kill, and chew the raw meat of animals. It is believed that primitive man initially was neither a hunter nor a gatherer; he fed on prey left by other truly carnivorous animals. Probably he did not even have the heartlessness required to attack and kill with his own hands innocent, unarmed, and peaceful animals.

26 Tannahill, R., 1995. Food in History. USA, Ney York, NY: Broadway

Perhaps, using sticks and stones, man was able to remove the antelope from the leopard and then would trail its body to his secure shelter. Such behavior is also known as profiteering.

But man did not just take away parts of the prey of carnivorous animals. He was also forced, when he had no chance of profiteering, to hunt directly, forcing in this way his natural non-aggressiveness due to the need of finding the means to survive.

Professor Facchini (professor of anthropology at the University of Bologna) says he is sure that prehistoric man worked the fire for culinary purposes, especially for cooking the meat. Also Professor Qakiaye Perles of the University of Paris agrees with this statement. Today, fortunately, there are no more cases of major force that forced our ancestors to feed on dead animals to make sure they had the necessary protein requirement. For a long time man has increasingly added to his own diet fresh fruits, vegetables, and greens.

However, we should always be careful and monitor the situation in order to defend ourselves from the ambush of food industries with their continuous proposals through propaganda via media and the evil work of mercenary doctors, as well as from substances that are of doubtful convenience or are even harmful.

HAVE WE BECOME CARNIVORES?

The man of the forest, where he lived for millions of years, had to move to the savannah. In the first era he was frugivorous, but in the savannah, given the lack of fruit, he had to become carnivorous.

Can it be that the human organism, as it was adapting to meat-based nutrition, adopted the anatomical and physiological characteristics typical of carnivores? No, it did not. Actually, it preserved the characteristics of a fruit-eating organism.

Today, after millions of years of unnatural meat nutrition, our nails did not turn into claws, our intestine did not shorten, our canine teeth did not elongate to become fangs, our gastric juices did not increase their original weak acidity typical of frugivores. The liver did not enhance its antitoxic ability, neither has the instinctive human attraction that makes humans prefer fruit during their childhood disappeared. And neither has the instinctive repulsion exerted by the child toward meat waned.

All these signs indicate that meat, despite all its negative characteristics and the enormous damages it has caused, failed to modify the physio-psychic structure of man. This proves that eating meat is so irrelevant to the nutritional and biological interests of man that he is not able to adapt to this type of nutrition in spite of having suffered the heavy consequences of an unnatural carnivorous instinct for a long time.

While I was writing this chapter, I heard a television report advertising the diet of the caves, i.e., that of our ancestors when they fed almost exclusively on meat. These gentlemen, together with a group of doctors, were trying to persuade viewers to switch to this diet because they thought it would be the most suitable for men. To be more convincing, they had come up with a nice novelty: according to them, thanks to the meat-based diet, our brain would develop and grow even three times more, passing from the 0.5 kg of brain of our ancestors to 1.5 kg of brain in man today. In other words, we have become the most intelligent species on Earth just because of eating meat.

Now I wonder: if man has become the most intelligent species on this planet only by eating meat, why then have carnivorous animals, considering that they do eat a lot more meat, not have evolved at least as much as we have done?

JEANNE CALMENT

Jeanne Louise Calment (February 21, 1875–August 4, 1997) was the longest-living human being for whom we have reliable information. She was born in Arles, France, and she lived 122 years and 164 days. I wanted to include her story in my book—even though I had available numerous other stories of super-centenarians who lived longer than she did—for the simple fact that her case is considered to be 100 percent certain. We have the confirmation of her birth. Such longevity was thoroughly documented by scientific studies on this case, and the verifying part required the deployment of means without precedence. In 1988, Guinness World Records assigned to her the record of the dean of humanity (although this does not mean that the other stories are not as truthful as hers).

      Jeanne Calment came from a long-living family. Her brother

lived 97 years, her father and mother lived 94 and 86 years respectively. When she was 21 years old, Jeanne married her second cousin Fernand Calment. Her lifestyle was very active, so active that she started to practice fencing at the age of 85. When she was 100 years old, she still rode a bicycle.

Jeanne came into the highlight of international news stories in 1988 when the centenary of the arrival of Van Gogh in her native city, Arles, attracted the media. This offered her the opportunity to speak with reporters.

Jeanne said she met Van Gogh when she was young. He asked her for money to help him paint. When journalists asked her about Van Gogh, she, who had met the painter when she was 13 in 1888, answered, "Ugly and hungry, but very kind to me. Despite being a shabby man consumed by alcohol, I gave him some money."

At the age of 114 years, Jeanne appeared shortly in the film *Vincent et moi* playing herself. This role also makes her the oldest actress ever. In 1995 a French documentary entitled *Beyond 120 years with Jeanne Calment* was published about her life.

This venerable French woman was born when the sky was plowed by air balloons, and she lived to the days when a wheeled robot traveled upon the surface of Mars. Nowadays, living a hundred years is almost trivial; at least this is what statistics say. But if we think about it, Jeanne Calment's longevity was not trivial. In her old age she was deaf and she mumbled her words. However, she saw her longevity with irony, "It's the fresh air that runs death away, and maybe the fact of having cycled until being a hundred years old."

HER SECRET

Some of her secrets were certainly physical activity and fresh air. We don't know much about her nutrition. All we know is that she ate little and her diet was rich in olive oil. Jeanne attributed her longevity and her relatively youthful appearance to this food, which she declared to have used in all types of food and even to spread it frequently on her skin. We know from her doctor that she had not been sick a single day in all her long life.

But what surprises us most is that she was a smoker. According to an unspecified source, Mme. Calment started smoking when she was 21 years old, but she wouldn't smoke more than two cigarettes per day. She stopped smoking when she was 117 years old, five years before her death.

It is terribly unfair, but it seems that there is a gene that protects some individuals against the damage caused by smoking. But how can it happen? So far, have I not argued that genes may have nothing to do with health? Don't worry, I was joking. A recent Russian survey conducted on long-living smokers showed—and the case of Jeanne Calment seems to confirm this hypothesis—that these people actually smoked only a little or they did not inhale the smoke. Certainly, smoking is a "secret" that should not be pursued. In any case, my point of view is that if Madame Calment had not smoked, she would have lived much longer.

The woman was also preserved by her nature, a positive attitude toward life, and an irrepressible sense of humor. In particular, she enjoyed the fact that she recorded her first album, a funk-rap called *The Lady of Time*, at the age of 120 years.

While carrying out research on the habits of those who have reached and exceeded one hundred years of age, I discovered something that applies to most of them: nearly all of them follow some regular and moderate physical activity that keeps them active. Among the popular activities there are cycling, walking, and gardening. Furthermore, these activities are not practiced to keep healthy, but for the simple pleasure of doing them.

In addition, all of these people maintained their irony, humor, and good moods, just as Mme. Calment did. All feel a lively interest toward the world around them.

Several studies have shown that pessimistic thinking favors the onset of diseases. One who sees everything as black needs more time to recover from an illness, and such a person is more prone to complications. Concentrating for a few minutes on a positive or negative event will cause our immune defenses to undergo changes.

PILLS: ELIXIR OF LONG LIFE?

"It lowers blood pressure." "It dissolves cellulite." "It reduces cholesterol." "It makes you lose weight." "It defends your heart." "It eliminates wrinkles." We can hardly resist such posts when we go to the supermarket and find them everywhere. Elixir here, elixir there. We turn on the television and there they are at any time of the day or night, promoted by accredited testimonials, to show us how to be deflated, how to pee more, how to take more calcium . . . and all of them, obviously, with zero calories!

We buy them and behold the miracle: the cellulite is gone, wrinkles disappear, the heart becomes stronger and we become younger and more beautiful. Am I right? I wish I were! On the contrary, everything is a lie. Why? Because pills do not constitute the source of health; rather, living foods do so, i.e., those foods that have not undergone any treatment, processing, or manipulation. Gandhi, in his book *Regime and Diet Reform*,[27] wrote, "To get rid of a disease, it is necessary to suppress the use of fire during the preparation of the meal."

Unfortunately, something new was born. It is called "Nutraceutical" and expresses a concept of nutrition as a medical aid, a clever mixture of food and medicine that creates products with hybrid characteristics between food and medicine. Too bad that science has nothing at all to do with these miraculous products.

The so-called "fat burning" pills consist, at best, of a combination of ingredients that have a high concentration of fibers, vitamins, and minerals. However, it has not yet been scientifically proven that this combination is able to block the absorption of fats. At best, these pills are a waste of money, says Erica Ilton, R. D., an expert on nutrition in New York.

Because these products are not regulated by precise rules, they might even be dangerous to our health, as confirmed by a recent study conducted by Swissmedic,[28] the Swiss institute for therapeutic agents. After analyzing 122 samples of "diet pills" in the laboratory—those best- known on the Internet—Swissmedic found that in nine out of ten cases the pills contained harmful substances. Some examples

27 Gandhi, M., 1949. *Diet and Diet Reform*. India, Ahmedabad: Navajivan Publishing House.

28 Media Release. June 6, 2011. "Alarming Analysis Results: Dangerous Slimming Products Available from the Internet: New Figures." Swiss Agency for Therapeutic Products [online].
Internet website:
http://www.swissmedic.ch/aktuell/00003/01658/index.html?lang=en

are sibutramine, withdrawn from the market more than a year ago all over the world, or rimonabant, a product that affects metabolism in different ways but does not produce any therapeutic benefit. In addition, the same research revealed that one third of the pills, although presented as purely herbal, contained chemical ingredients.

The amazing thing is that the food industry has put health-benefit indications on food labels for several years now. It is a pity that in 80 percent of the cases, the alleged health benefits listed on these food labels are based uniquely on the "scientific research" of profit.

The ones to certify this fact were experts of the NDA Panel of EFSA (European Food Safety Authority). These experts, based on an instruction of the European Commission, between 2008 and 2011 analyzed 2,758 food labels on nutrition and health in order to establish if there was solid scientific evidence behind their claims.

Experts rejected 80 percent of the entries on the labels because there were no serious studies that confirmed the health benefits, "The results of our research were favorable when there was sufficient evidence to support the claims. This was the case for about one out of five of the examined labels."[29] The press release can be read on the EFSA website in four languages: English, German, French, and Italian.

The latest episode was registered in the United States of America where an American court forced Ferrero Company to pay more than three million dollars for false advertising, because Nutella

29 Press Release. July 28, 2011. EFSA Finalizes the Assessment of "General Function" Health Claims. EFSA [online].
Internet website: http://www.efsa.europa.eu/en/press/news/110728.htm

was promoted as a "nutritious" and "healthy" product.

In 90 percent of the cases, food supplements, creams, elixirs, and all that comes from the "wellness industry;" are dangerous to our health, whereas the remaining 10 percent do nothing for us. The only thing that becomes thinner with these products is the buyer's wallet and health.

It is time to clear things: the only sure way of losing weight is healthy eating and more physical exercise. And, preferably, doing both things. I am not saying that we need to eat less, but that we need to eat healthy. The difference is subtle and it is about the diet we follow. The advice to eat less is true for all diets that use cooked foods, where a person can eat a lot in order to get very little. On the contrary, with the raw food diet we eat very little in order to get much.

CHAPTER 5

THE SUN:
THE UNKNOWN FOOD

Light is the primordial essence of the universe and all
life and movement derive from it. It is the Living and
Dynamic force of Nature.

Kabbalah

In this chapter we will talk about another food: the light of the sun.
According to the Kabbalah, light is seen as a kind of spiritual energy
beyond what we can perceive in this world through our senses. It
is the highest thing we can conceive. It is, in fact, a quality of the
Creator himself.

For those who do not know what the Kabbalah is, it is the
oldest and most mysterious form of wisdom of the world. It has
influenced philosophers, scientists, and great spiritual individuals of
all ages. We are born in the light, we live in the light, and we die in the
light. Everything is made of light. To better understand its enormous

rebalancing potential, consider that just the simple exposure to light produces beneficial effects on our bodies, our emotions, and our thoughts.

The human being is born to live in an environment illuminated by the sun and thus he can exploit the most potential when conducting a sunny lifestyle, i.e., with sufficient sunlight daily. Unfortunately, man is breaking this law.

It has been a long time now since we first heard negative things about the sun or, rather, of the harmful effects that sunlight has on humans. In particular, since the 1960s some scientific research has demonized the action of ultraviolet light. On the contrary, sunlight is real nourishment for our bodies and our being, so that poor lighting causes the same effects as poor nutrition.

This chapter will try to demonstrate, based on research, statistics, and rigorous scientific documentation, the positive effects of both sunlight and ultraviolet light either on human physiology or on the emotions. These researches have shown that the vast majority of ailments and health problems can be avoided or solved with a simple regular and correct exposure to sunlight.

The puzzling aspect is that despite the many scientific studies published almost all of the population is unaware of such information.

THE LIGHT

Light, as we know it, refers to the portion of the solar spectrum visible to the human eye. This portion, called the optical or the visible spectrum, coincides with that part of the solar spectrum that lies between red and violet and includes all the colors the human eye can see.

Therefore, just as the ear has its limits in the perception of sound, the human eye has its limits in the vision of light. In both cases, there are upper and lower limits, which may vary from person to person.

Conventionally, and just as an indication, it is possible to split the solar spectrum—electromagnetic spectrum—in various intervals or frequency bands, starting from the optical spectrum: cosmic rays, gamma rays, X-rays, ultraviolet radiation, visible light, infrared rays, microwave radiation, radio waves, acoustic waves, etc.

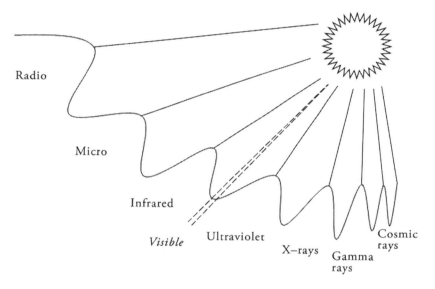

But this is not all. We also have dark energy and dark matter. The term "dark matter," which at first glance might seem mysterious, is simply the word that physicists, astrophysicists, and cosmologists give to the matter that does not emit visible light, radio waves, X-rays, gamma rays, or any other electromagnetic radiation. Today we know that the matter that emits some form of electromagnetic radiation— ordinary matter—constitutes only 4.6 percent.

The results from the WMAP satellite, dated back to 2008, that combined the data received from cosmic background radiation and other sources, indicate that the universe is composed of 72 percent dark energy, 23 percent dark matter, 4.6 percent ordinary matter, and less than 1 percent neutrinos.

The human visual system is able to transform and represent in colors only an extremely limited part of the visual waves that are within the ordinary matter. However, our body and all its cells perceive and react to all the other energies and forces of the universe.

ULTRAVIOLET RADIATION

Ultraviolet radiation (UV) is an electromagnetic radiation with a wavelength shorter than that of visible light but longer than x-rays. The name means "beyond violet" (from the Latin *ultra*, "beyond"), because purple is the color one can see with the shorter wavelength. When considering the effects of UV radiation on human health, the range of UV wavelengths is generally divided into:

UVA (400-315 nm)

UVB (315-280 nm)

UVC (280-100 nm)

The sun emits ultraviolet light in all three bands UVA, UVB, and UVC. Nevertheless, due to the absorption by the ozone layer, approximately 99 percent of the UV rays that reach the Earth's surface are UVA.

In fact, the atmosphere absorbs 100 percent of UVC and 95 percent of UVB rays. We should also consider that the normal glass of a window passes about 90 percent of light[30] that exceeds 350 nanometers and blocks 90 percent of the light below 300 nm. Therefore, glass lets in the UVA partially, while it shields almost totally against UVB and UVC.

THE MIRAGE

Man has always flattered himself with the idea of being able to see reality and has always considered reality what he could see and feel. But what we see and believe to be reality is just the interpretation and reconstruction of space in shapes and colors made by the visual cortex.

When our visual cortex transforms in colors the electromagnetic waves that affect the eyes, it does not mean that those waves or photons are the colors we see; rather, the human visual system attributes them such appearance to allow our minds to recognize them.

Color, therefore, is not a property of the matter. Simplifying, we could say that the matter we see has the property of absorbing ambient light of all wavelengths present in it, except for a few that are reflected and that our visual system can transform into what we believe to be the color of that matter. In other words, what we see and what we believe to be real is the result of "interpretations," "transformation," and "representations" of our brain of an extremely small part of the true reality made of energy, information, and energy interactions.

Thus, it is our brain that creates images, shapes, colors, and perspectives, which we believe to be the reality that surrounds us.

---

30 Sometimes, for simplicity, the word light is used more generally to identify all electromagnetic waves, i.e. even those invisible to the human eye.

However, our eyes perceive also all the other electromagnetic waves, such as ultraviolet or infrared rays, whose wavelengths are not transformed into shapes, colors, and images. They determine some reactions of the epiphysis (or pineal gland), the hypophysis (or pituitary gland), the hypothalamus, the entire endocrine and hormonal system, and the whole organism.

All electromagnetic waves, visible or not, determine energy and behavioral effects in all the structures of the matter with which they interact. Apart from the eyes and the visual system, our entire organism, every atom and every cell that constitutes it, responds and reacts to all wavelengths passing through it even if the visual system is not able to translate them into a visible form.

And what about artificial light? Does it produce the same effect on our bodies?

THE LIGHT WITHOUT LIGHT

A famous saying by Albert Einstein says, "Not everything that can be counted counts, and not everything that counts can be counted."

I was inspired by these words to formulate another saying: *Not everything that can light lights up, and not everything that lights can light up.* That is, not everything that can illuminate, such as traditional bulbs, really illuminates our bodies.

Many of the wavelengths in the solar spectrum linked to specific biological responses are not present in traditional lamps. Each of these wavelengths causes several effects and biological reactions. In artificial lighting when a specific wavelength or a group of wavelengths are absent, the body manifests disturbances. These disturbances can be more or less serious or evident due to the fact that, with regard to those wavelengths, it is the same as if the body was kept in darkness, even though other wavelengths are present.

In addition, not everything that illuminates[31] and really nourishes[32] our organism, such as ultraviolet or infrared rays, can be seen.

LAMPS

The traditional lamps used today for lighting—halogen, incandescent, or neon—although allowing us to see in the dark, produce just a limited spectrum of frequencies that are quite far from the sun. Furthermore, what unites all the artificial lighting produced for residential use is, in addition to the significant distortion of the frequency spectrum produced with regard to the sun, the elimination of ultraviolet rays that instead are necessary for human health. Artificial, traditional lighting, as we will see later, is harmful to either animals or plants.

Some lamp manufacturers, given the considerable difference between the sun and the emission spectrum of traditional lamps, began producing lamps with better emission characteristics. That is how full-spectrum, wide-spectrum, and ultraviolet light bulbs were born and can now be used in our houses. However, it is not easy to find them since they constitute a niche market. The wide-spectrum lamps are of higher quality than those of full spectrums. They are produced mostly in the United States. We cannot find them in common stores

---

31 As I said earlier, not being able to see certain electromagnetic waves with our eyes does not mean that they are truly invisible.

32 In addition to determining many physical and mental reactions, light nourishes our spirit and our vital energy.

or supermarkets, but we can easily buy them on the Internet.

Even if the source of artificial light could faithfully reproduce the emission spectrum of the sun, it cannot modify the spectrum in question dynamically during the day as the sun does.

SCIENTIFIC RESEARCH

Science has never been interested in the therapeutic or harmful effects of electricity, although it has made huge steps in technology since the light bulb was invented. The medical world has always greatly underestimated this aspect.

Lighting technology has developed artificial light based on the assumption of obtaining competitive ratios of brightness/power consumed. For producers, it is sufficient that artificial illumination makes it possible for us to see in the dark. All their studies are aimed at producing light sources that possess the characteristics of duration, consumption, power, dimensions, and emission areas able to satisfy every possible visual need. The spectrum of frequencies produced has always been compared to the chromatic visibility and the effects that certain frequencies can have on materials, rather than on the human body.

For the same power consumption, some wavelengths have a greater illuminating power. The ultraviolet and infrared, being invisible to the human eye, have no illuminating power. For this reason, artificial light is rich in some frequencies and lacks others that are important for our health.

Why has no one raised the issue of trying to imitate sunlight? The answer is that the lords of the lamps know they can get a white light that might have a similar appearance to that of the sun even with frequency spectra quite different from that of the sun. Therefore, they chose to combine together only those frequencies that have more illuminating power without limiting or obviously altering the vision of colors.

Just to give an example, the color blue, which is the frequency with the highest intensity in the solar spectrum, is also the least present in artificial light, given its illuminating power of only about five percent.

Conversely, the frequencies more common in artificial lighting such as red and yellow, which have a greater illuminating power, are those less present in the sun. Blue has a calming effect on the emotions and is characterized as calm and deep satisfaction. It produces an effect of quiet harmony. For the Chinese, blue is the color of immortality.

Red, however, has a stimulating effect, and it is not a coincidence that those who spend a lot of time under the light of the sun are, at a behavioral level, less stressed than those who live mainly with artificial lighting.

THE SUN

Every second the sun generates a large amount of electromagnetic radiation that makes life on Earth possible, providing the energy the Earth requires to activate its basic mechanisms. Furthermore, the insolation of the Earth's surface regulates the climate and most of the weather phenomena.

Man, and all forms of life on the planet, originated and

evolved as a result of exposure to sunlight. It has very specific characteristics, different from traditional artificial lighting, not only in terms of frequencies produced, but also in terms of daily and seasonal variability.

Artificial light is dull; its emission spectrum is always the same. Instead, the emission spectrum of solar energy reaching the Earth's surface changes dramatically from morning to night and from summer to winter, activating and stimulating endocrine and metabolic functions in different ways throughout the day and seasons.

Dr. J.N. Ott, one of the founders of photobiology and author of numerous publications on the therapeutic effects of light, writes in his book *Light, Radiation and You: How to stay healthy,*[33] "The human being has adapted himself to the complete emission spectrum of the sun. The artificial distortion of the spectrum leads to a bad illumination, a condition similar to malnutrition." During all his life, Dr. Ott has carried out important research on the effects of natural light on plants, animals, and humans.

Yet, before Dr. Ott, another German physician, C.W. Hufeland, in his 1796 manuscript *Macrobiotics or the Art of Prolonging Human Life,*[34] wrote, "The human being becomes pale, fat, lazy and apathetic and loses his vital energy if it is deprived of the sunlight, precisely as the sad observation of many prisoners locked up in the dark for long periods has shown."

---

33 Ott, J. N., 1985. *Light, Radiation, and You: How to Stay Healthy.* USA, Greenwich: Devin-Adair Pub.

34 Hufeland, C. W., 1796. Makrobiotik oder Die Kunst, das Leben zu menschliche verlängern. His manuscript has been translated into many languages, including Serbian in 1828.

CHANGING MENTALITY

The perception that the sun is harmful to our health is deeply rooted in our society. Most people look at the sun as something that is dangerous. This is the consequence of an erroneous education of the people arbitrarily planned by pharmaceutical companies to increase their benefits.

Perhaps few people know that in addition to the traditional scientific research, another one parallel to the first has been created sponsored by the multinational pharmaceutical, chemical, and food industries, a sort of pseudoscience that has been added and is unfortunately opposed to the true science. Its studies are based on the pursuit of the maximum profit. Everything bad that doctors have said against the sun in recent decades is a lie.

Another aspect that is important to take into consideration is that the positive effects described in this book, proved by true scientific research, have been often defamed by misleading information backed up by studies having a very different purpose, everything except searching for the truth.

These pseudoscientists, acting more because of greed and to defend their own economic interests, have introduced to medical and public opinion beliefs diametrically opposed to the truth. A feature of modern scientific research (pseudoscience) is to be able to show what you want or the opposite of what others have previously shown.

One should look to himself for the truth. We should not continue to believe only what someone else offers to us. It is useless to pretend that the results of an experiment are not affected by the objectives of those persons who lead and finance the experiment.

GUILTY OF INNOCENCE

The sun causes melanoma, cataracts, premature aging, degradation of the DNA, allergic reactions, and so on. So many accusations; and the sun cannot defend itself.

It is clear now that the sun and ultraviolet rays are used as a scapegoat by those trying to hide the real causes of the increase of tumors, of aging, or allergies. However, nobody dares attribute any responsibility to multinational corporations. Now it is time to stop believing all this nonsense. They are all lies!

In his book *The Influence of Ocular Light Perception on the Metabolism in Man and in Animal*, Professor F. Hollwich affirms,[35] "The natural light that involves the whole body is a vital element similar to water and air. Everyone should try to spend as many hours of the day outdoors as possible, according to the extent permitted by the seasons."

In the same book, Hollwich describes and presents numerous scientific studies that show how light affects the pineal gland, the endocrine system, growth and development, body temperature, water balance, red and white blood cell count, metabolization of fats, activity of the liver, levels of sugar in the blood, cortisol, ACTH, catecholamines, hormonal growth, etc.

Another important study by Beral et el, published in the prestigious scientific journal *Lancet*,[36] showed that rather than the

---

35 Hollwich, F., 1979, *The Influence of Ocular Light Perception on Metabolism in Man and in Animal*, Springer-Verlag.

36 Beral, V., Shaw, H., Evans, S., Milton, M., "Malignant Melanoma and Exposure to Fluorescent Lighting at Work," *The Lancet*, Vol. 320, Issue 8293, 7 August 1982, pp. 290–293.

sunlight, it is the light produced by fluorescent lamps which causes melanoma.

Considering a sample of 823 women, those exposed to fluorescent light showed a risk of melanoma more than two times higher than the others. The women showing the lowest risk were precisely the ones who were more exposed to sunlight. The risk of melanoma increased with the increasing duration of exposure to fluorescent light and it was greater in women who had worked mostly in offices.

LIES ABOUT EYEGLASSES

Another incredible and paradoxical aspect is that, according to baseless studies aimed at unleashing the population's fear of the sun and ultraviolet rays, the optical industry had to adapt itself quickly.

To prevent ultraviolet rays from reaching the eyes, sunglasses were imposed by law with the UV filter 400. In this way the ability for anyone to benefit from the positive effects of ultraviolet rays even when outdoors was further reduced.

In an article published in *Nexus Magazine*,[37] Joseph Hattersley reveals it is not true, as many ophthalmologists believe, that even low exposures to UVB rays can lead to an increased risk of developing cataracts. The disease is caused by junk food based nutrition, which is rich in saturated fats and oxidizing chemicals. In fact, those who eat properly, with fruits and vegetables, are not likely to develop cataracts even after long exposure to the sun.

---

37 Hattersley, J. G. "The Healing Power of Full-Spectrum Light," *Nexus Magazine*, Volume 8, Number 4.

Not only sunglasses, but also prescription eyeglasses reduce drastically the quantity of ultraviolet light that reaches the eyes. In fact, ultraviolet rays affecting the eyes regulate the proper functioning of certain endocrine and hormonal functions.

There is no doubt that sunglasses are a great invention that allows us to see better in environments with high brightness, such as in the mountains, for example. Today, however, sunglasses have become mainly a fashion and are used even when one can do without them. Eliminating the ultraviolet rays, even when we have those rare opportunities to be outdoors, is tantamount to depriving food to an already undernourished person.

Professor Jacob Liberman, with a doctorate in optometry and a Master's degree in vision science, and the author of numerous studies and texts, in his book *Light: Medicine of the Future*,[38] recommends spending at least an hour a day in plain air, whether there is bad weather or there is sun, without wearing glasses of any type, neither sunglasses nor prescription glasses, and without using sunscreens.

In his book *Health and Light*,[39] Dr. J.N. Ott explains how the body's chemistry and the metabolism of every cell and every tissue are influenced by the characteristics of the light entering the eyes and reaching the pineal gland.

Dr. Ott had a problem with hip arthritis that he could not treat in any way. This problem was preventing him from having a normal life. Although he had tried everything—diets, medications,

---

38 Liberman, J., 1991. *Light: Medicine of the Future*. USA, Santa Fe, NM: Bear & Company.

39 Ott, J. N., 1976. *Health and Light: The Effects of Natural and Artificial Light on Man and Other Living Things*. USA, Columbus, OH: Ariel.

warm baths, and other remedies—nothing seemed to work. Once, while he was in Florida for work, he decided to spend more time on the beach getting some sunshine. He knew that he could only benefit from the sun.

He did not notice any obvious benefit until one day he broke his eyeglasses, without which he could not do anything. Looking forward to the new ones, the doctor started using his spare ones, but they bothered his nose. So most of the time he began to be without glasses at all. Then the unbelievable happened; his pain began to decrease gradually.

Because he had tried everything to find a way to be healed from arthritis, he also considered the possibility that there might be a correlation with his eyeglasses. Although a few months before a doctor had offered him the possibility of hip surgery, a few months after he stopped wearing his eyeglasses, except when it was strictly necessary, Ott was healed.

People who have had problems such as osteoarthritis, arthritis, vision loss, diabetes, and even cancer, and have followed Ott's suggestion by trying to stay in the light of the sun as much as possible without glasses, have reported amazing benefits.

The lenses of eyeglasses, although transparent, induce a distortion in the wavelengths that can reach our eyes from the environment. Although in an invisible way, they eliminate almost completely the ultraviolet rays that affect the correct functioning of the delicate endocrine and hormonal systems.

In 1964[40] Dr. Ott was the first person to demonstrate that plants can reach their full development only if the sunlight comes to them without being reduced or distorted by any form of glass or transparent material.

Light entering the eyes must be as similar as possible to that of the sun. Anything that can change or distort it determines negative effects on the body. The richest season of ultraviolet rays is, of course, the summer. On a summer day, the highest concentration of rays is between nine in the morning and three in the afternoon, when 75 percent of the total rays reach the Earth. The peak hour, with about 20–30 percent of the total, is around noon. The clouds reduce the transmission of solar radiation on the Earth's surface, but the most that is reduced are visible light and infrared rays.

A LITTLE HINT

My recommendation for all those who wear eyeglasses is to try progressively not to use them, not only because they do not allow ultraviolet rays to reach the eyes but also because they make our sight worse.

Do not listen to the doctors who say that glasses are good for the eyes. Actually, glasses do well only to their pockets.

Eyesight can be cured definitively without glasses, laser, or surgery. Dr. Sidler-Huguenin, from Zurich, says[41] that the majority of

---

40 Ott, J. N., 1964. "Some Responses of Plants and Animals to Variations in Wavelengths of Light Energy." *Annals of the New York Academy of Sciences*, vol. 117, pp. 624–635.

41 Archiv. F. Augenh., vol. lxxix, 1915, translated in Arch. Ophth., vol. xlv, No. 6, 1916.

the thousands of myopics that he regularly treated got continuously worse in spite of his expertise in prescribing them the right eyeglasses to wear.

When eyeglasses break and we do not wear them for a week or two, sight improvement is often noticed. It is a fact that eyesight always improves when we eliminate the eyeglasses, although we do not always perceive it.

If we are really motivated to improve our eyesight, it just takes a little exercise and some movement. There are many natural ways to re-accustom the eye to see. One of these is the Bates method, developed by Dr. William Horatio Bates and published in his 1921 book, *The Cure of Imperfect Sight by Treatment Without Glasses*. This method aims to cure vision defects considered unsolvable—nearsightedness, farsightedness, presbyopia, astigmatism—through certain techniques and exercises. Dr. Bates believed that the use of glasses or surgery to correct vision problems was not only useless but also harmful. According to his research, all those who begin to use glasses will incur inevitable eyesight deterioration.

Despite the countless testimonies of healing through his method, it has never been recognized by traditional medicine. Do not forget that the eyewear industry is part of a huge global business.

Ophthalmologists know very well that eyesight tends to get worse if we use glasses, except that doctors are often remunerated in the form of commission on the glasses or the drugs that they sell. The conflict of interest is all too obvious. How do we know that our doctor does not prescribe a certain medicine just because that medicine assures him the best profit on the commission? We hear of such scandals every day.

For those who want to get out of this slavery, there are many books and DVDs on the market that teach us how to regain eyesight in a natural way.

WHEN IS SOLAR RADIATION HARMFUL?

It is said that when someone asked Leonid Brezhnev[42] which countries the Soviet Union bordered, he replied, "With all it wants to!"

In the healthcare industry, the matter is almost the same. People can be led to believe whatever the pharmaceutical industries want them to. They are masters at making healthy things appear harmful, and vice versa, with lots of scientific research and analysis to support what they teach. For example, there are "scientific researches" conducted on animals that have shown that ultraviolet rays are harmful.

An example is the ultraviolet-ray study carried out in 1981 by the Medical College of Virginia in Richmond by W. T. Ham and his colleagues.[43] In some anesthetized monkeys whose pupils were dilated and their eyes held open with retractors, after exposing the retina for a maximum of 16 minutes to 2,500 watt xenon lamps with high levels of ultraviolet radiation, damages to the retina were noted. Similar studies in which researchers burn the skin of laboratory animals with high levels of UV radiation are cited to show that UV light can cause skin cancer and cataracts.

---

42 Leonid Ilyich Brezhnev fue secretario del Partido comunista soviético de 1964 a1982.

43 Ham, W. T., et. al., "Action Spectrum for Retinal Injury from Near-Ultraviolet Radiation in the Aphakic Monkey," *American Journal of Ophthalmology*, March 1982.

These and other results along the same lines are being spread with such force in the world that they can convince everyone to banish UV rays from their lives. What is not being said, however, is that these experiments on animals are a real torture, with very high doses of radiation, unnatural and physiologically unmanageable.

In other words, it is as if someone wants to convince us that vitamins are noxious. This happens because, according to "scientific experiments," after administering to some monkeys "just" 250 grams of polar bear liver, rich in vitamin A, the monkeys died. Of course it is possible. But these "just" 250 grams contain 2,600 times the recommended daily dose. For a human being, just 100 grams of polar bear liver would be enough to put an end to his life.

A well-known nutritionist, Basil Brown, decided to drink several liters of carrot juice every day in order not to grow old and to remain always young. What were the consequences? Ten days later he died of intoxication from vitamin A! In fact, carrot juice contains 80 percent of beta-carotene, which later turns into vitamin A. Can we therefore deduce that vitamin A or other vitamins are noxious? Yes, we can. If vitamins are taken in unnatural and physiologically unmanageable quantities, they are noxious . . . just as in the case of the experiment with 2,500 watt lamps.

Another very underestimated aspect of scientific research is that the obtainable results depend to a great extent either on the type of light that is used or on the initial conditions of the experimentation subjects. If we want to demonstrate the negative effects of exposure to ultraviolet light, it is sufficient to use for the experiment people who are very deficient in UV and who are used to an oxidizing nutrition.

It is said that where there is a will, there is a way. And pharmaceutical companies know that very well. They just need to want to demonize some essential element for human health in order to see increases in their economic power.

Even water, if you think about it, can be harmful if taken in large quantities and all at once. The same also applies to the healthiest foods. This reminds me of an incident that happened when I was still in college. A student bet that he would be able to drink five liters of water in five minutes. He made it, but it nearly cost him his life. He had water intoxication.

If we jump from a height which is less than two meters, probably our muscles will bear it. But if we jump from a height of twenty meters, death will be almost inevitable. And so, once again, is jumping dangerous? Yes, it is. No, it is not . . . Well, it depends.

MELANOMA

In recent years, a massive campaign of media terrorism has emphasized the dangers of exposure to sunlight, especially in relation to skin cancer, namely melanoma. Melanoma is a type of skin cancer which owes its name to the special skin cells called melanocytes. It may be fatal if it is not treated properly and promptly. However, numerous scientific studies have demonstrated that the sun not only is not responsible for the increasing incidence of melanoma, but instead reduces it.

The diffusion of such terror, basically false, has given the pretext to create a new large market: chemical sunscreens. For the manufacture of such products, anything except harmless substances are used. Most of the chemicals found in sunscreens, in fact, are toxic and increase the risk of developing cancers, and not just skin cancers. Furthermore, many of them cause mutations in the DNA as a result of their interactions with the light at cellular levels.

At the same time, public attention is diverted to a culprit that cannot defend itself—the sun—allowing the chemical industry to continue increasing its benefits undisturbed.

For millions of years man has lived in nature, depending on it. He followed and respected nature. He adapted himself to its cycles and is elements, receiving from it life and energy.

Nowadays, a general weakening is evident. Diseases and ailments that did not exist before now appear daily. And what the medicines of today do, unfortunately, is to suppress the symptoms and to create the need of follow-up treatment.

Healing goes against the interests of those who produce the medical treatments and who need regular and constantly growing consumers. A clear example that disproves the alleged harmful effects of the sun and ultraviolet rays in relation to melanoma is that the incidence of melanoma, and of deaths related to it, is higher in the northern countries. It decreases progressively as we move toward the south where populations are more exposed to sunlight.

If the primary cause was really the sun, then the opposite should be true. From this example we can easily deduce that the sun not only does not cause melanoma, but rather it fosters our protection, reducing the risk of cancer.

In 1970, Professor Howard Maibach showed that more than 35 percent of sunscreen applied to the skin enters the bloodstream when exposed to the sun.[44] In addition, the absorption of chemicals is greater if they remain longer on the skin. Not surprisingly, the incidence of skin cancer in the world has grown in direct proportion to the use of sunscreens.

According to Dr. Gordon Ainsleigh, in a study published in *Preventive Medicine* magazine,[45] "the use of sunscreens causes more cancer and deaths than those which they should theoretically prevent." Dr. Ainsleigh has estimated that 17 percent of lung cancers observed between 1981 and 1992 may have been related to the massive use of sunscreens in the past ten years.

DO NOT PUT EVERYTHING UNDER THE SAME UMBRELLA

What creates more confusion about UV rays is the tendency of the press to put all kinds of ultraviolet rays under the same umbrella.

Actually, as we mentioned earlier, there are three types of ultraviolet rays: UVA, UVB and UVC. So far we have spoken only of the first two, UVA and UVB rays, the ones that reach the Earth.

The rays to which we must pay more attention are indeed the UVC, the ones with the highest energy. This type of UV radiation has a bactericidal and germicidal action. Due to their high energy that can damage the tissues, they are used to kill bacteria and viruses.

We should give special attention to these types of UV rays because the exposure to even a very low intensity can cause damage

---

44 Maibach, H., 19 May, 1978. NDELA-Percutaneous Penetration. *FDA* Contract 223-75-2340.

45 Ainsleigh, H. G., January 1993, "Beneficial Effects of Sun Exposure on Cancer Mortality," *Preventive Medicine*, Vol. 22, pp. 132–140.

to us. This could happen, for example, if we expose ourselves to a sunlamp with damaged filters or a lamp used for sterilization. Some might find themselves exposed to the action of these rays, even at high doses, without even realizing it, and consequently suffer the damage.

With regard to the sun, do not worry since the UVC rays are completely absorbed by the atmosphere.

TWO INSEPARABLE FRIENDS

In order to fully enjoy the benefits of the sun, it is important to follow a natural diet. With natural diet I mean eating only those foods that are not processed or treated in any way, i.e., raw foods.

Dr. Zane Kime, in his book *Sunlight Could Save Your Life*,[46] explains the concept clearly. "If a person does not follow a proper diet, sunlight can have adverse effects. I have to emphasize this fact: sunbathing is dangerous for people with a nutrition like the average diet in the United States, with high fat concentration and low concentration of vegetables, cereal and fresh fruit. They must avoid the sun and protect themselves from it. And they will suffer the consequences of both poor nutrition and lack of sunlight."

Sun exposure could be risky in only two cases. First, when the body does not receive adequate food rich in enzymes, antioxidants, and vitamins, and when it is not well hydrated. Second, the rays can hurt us when we expose ourselves to the sun for hours immediately after spending months in an office with neon lights, not allowing our organism to be prepared to handle such energies. It is the same as giving a sumptuous meal to a seriously undernourished person. That

---

46 Kime, Z.R., 1980. *Sunlight Could Save Your Life*. USA, Pinryn, CA: World Health Publications.

person, in fact, after a meal like that might even die. For example, it is well known that when you restart eating after a long fast you should be very careful. First of all, you need to allow the digestive system to restart functioning little by little.

The same applies to sunlight. After being forced during the whole year to deprive ourselves of exposure to sunlight in rooms with artificial, limited, and distorted lighting, in the summer when we expose ourselves to the sun for the first time we are totally unprepared because we come from a situation of serious deficiency of sunlight.

To make things even worse, we have an unnatural nutrition rich in chemicals such as preservatives, pesticides, food colorants, and many others. All of them have an oxidant action on our organism.

When the body is prepared, it can easily handle all radiation without problems. I've watched my father's behavior since I was a child. When spring arrives, he starts to work in the garden. As the temperature increases, he takes off more pieces of his clothing until he wears just shorts. So, when summer arrives, he is already tanned and prepared. During the summer he can sunbathe all day, at any time and temperature, without getting burnt or suffering any damage. And my father does not make the exception. Everyone in the country where I grew up follows this kind of solar lifestyle.

When I was a child, neither my brothers nor I, nor the friends with whom we used to play all day in the sun, ever reported problems caused by the sun. The problem with the sun never existed and we did not even know about it.

During all my life, I have never used any sunscreen because where we were living sunscreens were considered a strange fashion and even a stupid one. On a subconscious level, we knew that making use of them was a big mistake.

We had noticed these things in our cousins who lived in the city. When they used to come to spend the summer with us in the countryside, they seemed like chickens that just went out of their incubators or cages. They were very pale and anemic.

My aunt, owner of a big pharmacy, used to give them lots of drugs and vitamins. Nevertheless, I always remember their having colds and being sick. They were thin and weak, almost like the starving children of Africa except that unlike the latter ones, my cousins did not lack anything apart from the sun and proper nutrition. Their mother always advised them to stay out of the sun. If for some reason they wanted to expose themselves to the sun, they had to put on sunscreen. Or, if the children wanted to eat fruits or vegetables picked from our garden, first of all they had to wash it thoroughly, otherwise they were at risk of getting sick because of the parasites and germs contaminating the fruits.

In our family we always ate only fruits, vegetables, and greens from our own garden. The reason was not that we knew those on the market were treated with pesticides and other chemical substances, but that it was a custom handed down from my grandparents.

As a child, when I used to go to our garden, in spite of all the germs that unwashed fruits and vegetables could have, I simply picked up some of them as they were, dirty with germs, and ate them without even washing them. I must say that none of us ever suffered any ailments due to these elusive germs. It is clear that the fear induced by the chemical industry against germs is just another of the many pretexts to increase their profits.

SOME BENEFITS OF THE SUN

All the positive effects listed below have been documented and proven by many rigorous and indisputable scientific studies. The sun:

1) activates the synthesis of vitamin D3 for the absorption of calcium;
2) improves development and growth;
3) reduces the formation of dental cavities;
4) increases resistance against diseases, including tumors;
5) improves the efficiency of the cardiovascular system;
6) reduces blood pressure;
7) reduces cholesterol levels in the blood;
8) improves mental performance and learning skills;
9) regulates the sleep-wake cycle;
10) improves osteoarthritis, arthritis, and rheumatism;
11) improves eyesight;
12) improves all the endocrine and hormonal functions;
13) has an aesthetic function (tan);
14) increases testosterone (male) and progesterone (female) levels;
15) improves the emotional state and fights depression;
16) regulates alkalinity in the blood;
17) has a germicidal and prophylactic effect against infectious diseases;
18) stimulates metabolism and contributes to weight loss;
19) has a positive effect in the treatment of asthma, airways, and tuberculosis;
20) extends life.

AN ENDLESS LIST

To be able to describe all the benefits that derive from sunlight, we should write at least a dozen books. In the same way, dozens of other books should be written in order to list only the damages caused by artificial light or lack of exposure to sunlight. Therefore, what you read in this chapter is nothing more than an attempt to summarize, at least in part, what I have considered fundamental. Those who wish to further investigate this issue will certainly find on the Internet or in bookstores many scientific papers on the benefits of the sun. The important thing is to choose the right books.

WIDE-SPECTRUM LAMPS

I recommend to all those persons who, due to business or other reasons, cannot be exposed sufficiently to sunlight, to install at home, in their office, and in the places where they spend a lot of time, wide-spectrum and ultraviolet light sources. At the moment, it seems that the best light sources are the American Lumichrome® ones. All the information needed about them can be found on the Internet.

SARHAT RASHIDOVA

Sarhat Rashidova (1875–September 16, 2007), was born in Zidyan, a small village near Derbent, in the Republic of Dagestan. She passed away while she was sleeping at her children's house on September 16, 2007.

Sarhat never knew her parents and was raised by her grandparents. She married late to a widower with five children from his previous marriage, four boys and one girl.

Sarhat had no children of her own. She raised and looked after those of her husband, who died in the 1950s. She continued working until a few years before passing away. "We had a very demanding mother, and we are so grateful to her," said Gadzhifeti Karimov, 86-years old and the youngest of the adopted children of Sarhat, during a television interview in 2007.

The confirmation of the longevity of this lady comes from her passport. The chief of police of Derbent describes how, by chance, he happened to find her passport:

"In 2003, we substituted our old Soviet passport with the Russian one. The family brought me Sarhat's passport. *Is there a mistake?* I wondered. At first I could not believe it. I knew she was old. I had known her for about 40 years and I always remembered her having been like that. Her appearance had not changed at all. However, I could never imagine that she was so old. We did not believe the fact until an investigation confirmed Sarhat's real age."

Sarhat lived almost her entire life in a house made of clay. She had Azeri origins and spoke only Azerbaijani. She witnessed the happening of historical events such as the death of Tsar Alexander II of Russia during a terrorist attack; the ascendance of Alexander III; the killing of the last tsar of the Romanov dynasty, Nicholas II, in 1918; and the end of the Soviet Union in 1991. She also witnessed the Bolshevik Revolution, as well as the First and Second World Wars. In 1940, together with many other people from Dagestan, Sarhat dug anti-tank trenches around Derbent and Makhachkala to prevent the advance of the German army.

The climate in the region of Derbent is considered one of the most favorable, since it is located on a plain near the mountains and the sea. According to some specialists, the Caucasus Mountains were home to some of the longest-living people in the world. Due to their geographical isolation and ancient customs, her home area was a perfect antidote for anxiety and stress.

According to her friends and family, Sarhat never suffered

from any disease nor complained of any pain. She never made use of medicines nor alcohol. During her last years of life, she worked in a kolkhoz (agricultural cooperative) where without help she cared for four cows in addition to chickens and geese.

Her relatives tried several times to bring Sarhat to live with them in the city, but every time she went back home. In an interview, while she was staying in Dagestanskiye at the home of one of her sons, she said, "I made it to stay in the city for a month, at most. It is definitely not a place for me. In the city," she complained, "the air is bad and I want to go home."

At the beginning in Zidyan there were 180 families, but most of them are gone now. All of her children, grandchildren and, great-grandchildren, 62 in total, moved to the cities and major villages. For many years Sarhat lived alone in Zidyan.

Her family says that she was always an optimistic person. She never complained about the difficulties of life, family tragedies, and never suffered from loneliness. Sarhat used to participate and dance happily in all country festivals. She was highly motivated and made recommendations to her grandchildren till the end of her days.

Sarhat used to begin the morning with a prayer and then it was time to feed the poultry. After that she normally ate breakfast, took care of the garden and did the housecleaning. She almost always had something to do and was never idle.

In the village, everyone loved her for her kindness. Mardan, her 80-year-old neighbor, said, "When I was little, she used to hold me in her arms and to feed me with milk, eggs, and biscuits."

The granny Sarhat did not know the secret of her longevity. The leader of the village of Zidyan says, "I think I know her secret. Since I remember her, she was always welcoming and kind. When we were still children and used to go to her house to visit her, she always gave us lots of things to eat. But this is not all. I think that the clean air, spring water, and the fact that everything here is natural have contributed as well."

SARHAT'S SECRET

Undoubtedly, there are many factors that contributed to the longevity of Sarhat. Optimism, serenity, and vitality are just some of them. She liked to work and help others. She never felt useless. She always prayed and had faith in God. Surely, the environment helped with her longevity too.

She ate only food from her garden. Her diet consisted mainly of milk, eggs, fruits, and vegetables of her own production.

The night before she died, Sarhat said she was feeling well. And then she fell asleep, passing away while sleeping.

Another thing that unites these long-living persons is that all of them spent many hours in the sunlight and fresh air, working and taking care of their gardens.

IS CHOLESTEROL HARMFUL?

There is a lot of misinformation about cholesterol. Contrary to popular belief, cholesterol is an essential nutrient for our organism. The brain, for example, needs it in large quantities. As a matter of fact, the brain consists of cholesterol in a percentage that shifts from 10 to 20 percent.

Cholesterol also:

- ✓ is involved in the formation and repair of cell membranes;
- ✓ helps regulate the exchange of nutrients and waste products across the cell membrane;
- ✓ is the precursor of steroid hormones and sex hormones (such as androgens, testosterone, estrogen, and progesterone);
- ✓ is a constituent of pituitary, adrenaline, and gonadal hormones;

✓ is contained in hemoglobin;

✓ is the precursor of bile salts;

✓ is converted into vitamin D when exposed to ultraviolet light from the sun;

✓ helps insulate nerve fibers;

✓ acts as a conductor of nerve impulses;

✓ protects against infection;

✓ extends life.

Most of the cells of our body can produce the cholesterol which is not present in food. However, many people, as soon as they hear the word "cholesterol," seriously fear that they will die prematurely of a heart attack.

Hypercholesterolemia was practically unknown until 30 years ago. But within a short time, for tens of millions of people around the world, it switched to the top of the list of concerns about their health.

Nowadays, measuring cholesterol levels has become a popular pastime. Certain doctors and certain pharmaceutical companies are doing their best to encourage this new hobby. The reason is, of course, that they can make great profits from it.

Cholesterol has gained a bad reputation because of its association—which of course is false—with the rise in cardiovascular diseases. In fact, the viewpoint that high cholesterol is the cause of serious health problems is not based on evidence, but rather on clues, many of which are proved to be groundless when checked.

In 1953 Ancel Keys, a researcher at the University of Minnesota, published a study that would become the founding myth of the theory on cholesterol. In the study, the author inserted a diagram based on the assumption that, in six different countries worldwide, he found a clear relationship between fat consumption and mortality due to coronary heart diseases.

The curve of the diagram still causes a big impression. It is, however, based on a limited amount of data. In fact, when drawing it, Keys took into consideration only data related to six countries in the world, despite having available the figures for 22 countries. If he had used all the available data, he would have seen that the relationship between fat consumption and death due to heart attacks proves to be nonexistent.

"If only Keys had included in his research all the countries whose data were available, he could not have drawn that curve in his diagram," says the Swedish doctor Uffe Ravnskov. "For example, in the United States, mortality from coronary heart disease was three times higher than in Norway, although in both countries the consumption of fat was roughly the same."

The large-scale programs aimed at educating people are false when they lead us to believe that the theories on cholesterol in fashion today are a reality taken for granted in the medical field.

In many pharmacies there are, for example, brochures available to customers where they can read sentences such as, "Starting from your thirties, you should know your cholesterol level and check it every two years." Another example is, "Cholesterol is a time bomb for your health."

The principle that they want to make us believe as true is that hypercholesterolemia is "one of the most frequent risk factors" for heart disease.

Paul Rosch, president of the American Institute of Stress and professor of medicine at the New York Medical College, declares, "The brainwashing of the public opinion has worked so well that many people believe to be healthy and to live longer is to have a low cholesterol rate. On the contrary, there is nothing more erroneous than this belief."

Who are the main slanderers of cholesterol? Certainly, we can identify those who gain some kind of benefit from its defamation. And there are plenty of them. The health initiatives regularly organized by the Federal German cardiologists, the Becel enterprise, the Pfizer pharmaceutical group and the Roche Diagnostics enterprise, are just some of the many outstanding examples. Their goal is to convince people to measure the cholesterol level in their blood.

In 2001, over a million people who were concerned about their cholesterol levels, were tested during health campaigns. As one might expect, it was found that in more than half of the people examined, cholesterol levels were above the threshold arbitrarily set at 200.

So cardiologists have new patients who visit them. And they advise their patients not to eat butter. This is, of course, good news for Becel, a producer of margarine. Pfizer, instead, earns billions of Euros selling drugs worldwide that reduce cholesterolemia. In addition, Roche Diagnostics produces equipment for measuring the cholesterol level. Meanwhile, doctors and drug companies are getting rich.

Very seldom have we seen an advertising campaign that induces the majority of the population to consider themselves sick organized with such conviction and such waste of resources. And behold the coup de théâtre: people with high cholesterol are those who live longer than others.

Having been brainwashed, this statement may seem so incredible that we need a long time to assimilate it and to fully understand its importance. Yet the fact that individuals with a high cholesterol level may live longer emerges clearly through many scientific studies.

Let us consider the 1994 results of Dr. Harlan Krumholz of the Cardiovascular Medicine Department at Yale University. He revealed that among older people who had a low cholesterol level the mortality rate recorded was twice as high due to heart attacks than among the elderly who suffered from high cholesterol.[47] Campaigners in favor of low cholesterol remain consistent with their perspective and simply ignore this objection or consider it as a rare exception that happens only randomly, despite the fact that there are a large number of studies supporting the contrary.

This is not an exception, however. At present, there are a multitude of researches available that contradict the lipid hypothesis. In the present case, numerous studies on older people have shown that high cholesterol is not a risk factor for coronary heart disease. This is the result of research conducted by Dr. Uffe Ravnskov and published in the Medline database.[48]

Eleven studies conducted on elderly people led to the above result. Another seven studies have found that a high cholesterol level is not an all-comprehensive predictor of mortality.

47 Krumholz, H. M., et al "Lack of Association Between Cholesterol and Coronary Heart Disease Mortality and Morbidity and All-Cause Mortality in Persons Older Than 70 Years." *Journal of the American Medical Association*, 272(17):1335–1340, November 2, 1994.

48 Ravnskov, U "High Cholesterol May Protect Against Infections and Atherosclerosis." *Quarterly Journal of Medicine*" 96, 2003, pp. 927–934.

Now, consider that more than 90 percent of all cardiovascular diseases are present in people who are more than 65 years old, and almost all the studies have shown that a high cholesterol level is not a risk factor. This implies that high cholesterol constitutes a risk factor of less than five percent among those who die of a heart attack.

And there is a further reassuring thing for those who have high cholesterol: six studies have revealed that total mortality is inversely related to total cholesterol, or to LDL cholesterol, or to both of them. Therefore, if we want to live for a long time, actually it is much better to have a high cholesterol level rather than a low one.

There are many studies that indicate that a low cholesterol level is, in some respects, worse than a high level. For example, in 19 large studies involving more than 68,000 deceased patients examined by Professor David R. Jacobs and his colleagues of the Division of Epidemiology at the University of Minnesota, it was found that low cholesterol suggests an increased risk of death due to gastrointestinal and respiratory diseases.[49]

Most of gastrointestinal and respiratory diseases have an infectious origin. An important question at this point is whether it is the infection which lowers the cholesterol or if a decreasing level of cholesterol makes a way for the infection.

In order to answer this question, Professor Jacobs and his team, together with Dr. Carlos Iribarren, for 15 years monitored more than 100,000 individuals with good health in the San Francisco

---

49 Jacobs, D., et al.,. "Report of the Conference on Low Blood Cholesterol: Mortality Associations." Circulation 86, 1992, pp. 1046–1060.

area.[50] At the end of the study, it turned out that individuals who had a low cholesterol level at the beginning of the study had been hospitalized more often than others as a result of infectious diseases. We cannot object to such results claiming that it was the infection which reduced the cholesterol since the measurements showed that cholesterol was already low when the subjects had no evident infection. Instead, it seems that the low cholesterol, in some way, made people more exposed to infection or, in other words, that high cholesterol protected those who did not have infections.

In the book *The Cholesterol Myths*,[51] Dr. Uffe Ravnskov shows that people who by nature have a high cholesterol level (in medicine this case is known as family hypercholesterolemia) are protected from infection. If being born with high cholesterol protects against infection, then being born with low cholesterol should have the opposite effect. And indeed, this seems to be the case.

Children affected by Smith-Lemli-Opitz syndrome have a very low cholesterol level because the enzyme needed for the last step of the synthesis of cholesterol in the organism does not work as it should. The majority of children with this syndrome are born dead or die a short time after birth due to severe malformations of the central nervous system. Children who survive have mental retardation and an extremely low cholesterol level. Furthermore, they are affected by frequent and severe infections. However, if their diet is complemented

---

50 Iribarren, C., et al., 1997. "Serum Total Cholesterol and Risk of Hospitalization, and Death from Respiratory Disease," *International Journal of Epidemiology*, Vol. 26, pp. 1191–1202.

51 Ravnskov, U. *The Cholesterol Myths: Exposing the Fallacy That Saturated Fat and Cholesterol Cause Heart Disease*. USA, Washington, DC: New Trends Publishing, 2002.

with pure cholesterol or with the addition of eggs, their cholesterol level rises and they are less susceptible to infections.

If we were to follow the advice of some doctors regarding cholesterol, we should not even feed infants with breast milk because it is a real source of cholesterol.[52] But, in reality, children fed with their mother's milk are those who grow healthier. This is not surprising, considering that in order to be structured, nerve cells and the brain need the abundant cholesterol contained in breast milk.

Statins are medicines that inhibit the synthesis of endogenous cholesterol. Such property makes them to be a product of fundamental importance for the pharmaceutical industry. Individuals who may need statins are many, i.e., all those whose cholesterol level has been defined as too high and therefore are really in need of treatment. They do not have other problems except a high cholesterol level. They are in good health and thus are likely to live long enough to need to take statins every day for decades.

As a matter of fact, the substances that prevent the formation of cholesterol have proved themselves to be great money makers in the market of pharmaceutical products. They are protected by patents and can be purchased only at a high price (approximately from one to two Euros per daily dose).

Pfizer expects to reach an annual turnover of ten billion dollars thanks only to the production of a statin called Lipitor. Today, Lipitor is the best-selling pharmaceutical product of all time. The statin produced by its competitor Merck & Co., named Zocor, reaches

---

52 The content of cholesterol in breast milk is three times higher than that of cow's milk.

no less than the staggering amount of $7.5 billion. In the United States, 5.4 percent of the adult population take statins regularly; in the world there are 44 million consumers. The sale of these drugs has skyrocketed in the last decade because the number of people classified as suffering from high cholesterol has increased excessively.

As it happens in the case of many other diseases, the definition of high cholesterol is reviewed periodically. In the same way, as with other pathologies, such definition has been enlarged in order to include and classify as sick an increasing number of healthy people.

With the passage of time, the boundaries that define a disease gradually expand, and the group of potential patients is constantly expanding. Sometimes the increase is unexpected and striking. Some years ago in the United States, a committee of "experts" on cholesterol reformulated their definitions. Among other changes they made, they decided to lower the cholesterol levels considered necessary to authorize a medical treatment. Basically, the new definition classified as sick millions of healthy people and almost tripled overnight the number of individuals who could be subject to drug therapy.

On the contrary, all the diseases attributed to cholesterol are due to a poor diet, lack of physical exercise, poor exposure to sunlight, the use of various medicines, and many other causes.

CHAPTER 6

HOW DO WE LIVE TODAY?

The duration of human life depends on many factors. One
of these is, no doubt, the environment in which people live.

Dr. A. Petroff

In biology, the word *environment* indicates anything that can directly
affect the metabolism or the behavior of an organism or living species,
including light, air, water, soil, and other living things.

If the quote by Dr. A. Petroff somehow discourages a person
because he thinks he is not part of those few lucky persons who live in
the best areas of this planet that are good for human longevity, know
that there is an old saying that says, "It's not the place; it's the people."

This means that man alone can, to a large extent, create
the necessary conditions he needs to live. For example, when our
ancestors had to leave their villages because there was a lack of space
or resources, the first thing they did was to look for new territories,

new habitats. But even when they found one, it was certainly not a welcoming place. It was desolate, primitive, and unsuited to their needs. At that point they knew that if they wanted to survive they had to build houses, plant trees, grow crops, etc. In some way, they had to tame and humanize that territory. It reminds me of an episode during my adolescence when I was about 14 years old. I went on a trip with my classmates. We had to hike 90 km. We all armed ourselves with food, water, tents, and everything else that was needed for our survival because we had to sleep in the open air. It was a fantastic experience that I would recommend to anyone.

The route was circular, so at the end of the 90 km we would return to the starting point. Everybody had binoculars, maps, and compasses in their hands. We crossed forests, valleys, mountains, and rivers. Everything was far from residential areas.

We were organized for everything we needed. Nothing was lacking, not even music. We had brought with us almost all the necessary tools that would help us transform and create our perfect environment. We were doing exactly as our ancestors had done thousands of years before. In fact, the trip was really intended that way. It was a survival trip.

DIFFERENT ENVIRONMENTS

Although in theory all of us had the same equipment, each of us was also free to carry things that he thought were the most appropriate for survival. For example, among all of us there was only one girl carrying mosquito spray. Needless to say, thanks to that spray our classmate had guaranteed for herself an environment free of mosquitoes. On the contrary, I was standing a meter away from her in an environment that was full of mosquitoes that did not stop stinging me.

Or, for example, two boys had brought with them some small equipment for fishing. There was also someone who had covertly brought some cigarettes. These are just a few examples because, of course, everyone had brought with them different things depending on what they considered necessary.

The same thing happens even at a family level. Each member has a particular lifestyle. For example, one prefers to sleep with the window open during the night, while another prefers the window closed. Someone likes hot food, whereas someone else likes room temperature or cold food. So even if they live in the same house, two people can live in different environments. Wherever we are, all of us are free to choose in which environment to live.

ENVIRONMENT AND LONG LIFE

Certainly the quality of life has dramatically improved over the last hundred years. This phenomenon has coincided with the Industrial Revolution and technological progress, which led to the fact that the living conditions of the population have improved considerably. The progressive increase in the duration of life is the most important phenomenon of our time, especially in industrialized countries. It is, of course, due to the achievements in the medical field, but not only that; to a greater degree it is also due to environmental improvements and thus to technological, social, and economic progress. The latter type of progress has enabled man to avoid some of the most exhausting work and has also allowed the elderly to live in better environments.

I am referring to running water and heat, for example, that have been fundamental achievements during the last century.

In developing countries, we find a limited number of individuals over 100 years of age. But in 2050 their share will rise to 50 percent of the total, since needed improvements will become important in those areas.

Then there are those super-centenarians who were able to take advantage of favorable environmental conditions or who adopted sober lifestyles. Although they lived in poor or developing countries, they enjoyed a less polluted environment. Many of them ate products coming mainly from their organic gardens situated on land that had not yet been polluted by the chemical industry.

IN JESUS' TIME

The chemical, pharmaceutical, and food industries justify themselves by declaring that one or two thousand years ago the earth and the food were not chemically treated yet life expectancy was much lower than today. They claim that food manipulation is not harmful to our health, but rather improves it given that the average length of life has doubled since then. This is true, especially in the last hundred years with the advent of the Industrial Revolution.

Nevertheless, this claim is not totally correct. In fact, we have already seen that it has been possible to improve life thanks to technological, social, and economic progress.

For example, we had to wait until 1855 before we could use the heaters invented by the Italian-Russian Franz Karlovich Sangalli. Before that time, people were forced to endure great discomfort and

155

cold in the winter, considering that only one room or two were heated. This is one reason why people got sick more easily.

Colds, bronchitis, and pneumonia were only a few of the diseases from which people were dying at that time. And all this took place by the light of candles; the light bulb did not exist yet. We had to wait until 1880 for its invention.

In any case, for the heater and the light bulb to be spread in the market took another 30 years. From the invention or the registration of a patent to the expansion of the product at a national or global level takes several years.

And what about the refrigerator, small electrical appliances, the radio, the TV, and computers? All of them have contributed to the improvement of our economy, information, education, and many other aspects of our lives.

Today when we go to buy fruits and vegetables, we do not even notice that they come from the most diverse places in the world. If we had to go personally to collect these foods, each of us should have to travel several thousand kilometers. Just to name a few, we can think of bananas from Ecuador, kiwi from Italy, oranges from the USA, grapefruit from South Africa, etc. Our ancestors certainly did not have this possibility.

FOOD PROCESSING AND COOKING

Now we have to face another issue that is not of a lesser relevance. I am talking about the processing and cooking of foods. We all know that now, more than ever, our food is processed and refined. Among the best-known processed foods are sugar, bread, and oil. These are only a few of them.

A question naturally arises, why do we do it? Or, more precisely, why do they do it? This is a good question. First of all, they do it to make the food appear more appetizing, thus leading us to buy it. Second, they do it for their economic benefit.

Formerly sugar was brown, but now it is white. Bread was black and compact, whereas now it is white and fluffy. Oil was more consistent and flavorful, while now it is more fluid and smooth.

Nowadays infants, and many adults as well, do not know the true color and flavor of many foods because everything is colored and flavored. It is obvious that many children have a wrong idea about food.

If by chance we were faced with a natural product, we would probably think it was not natural. For example, the vivid pink color of some species of fish, such as trout or salmon, in reality should be less colored. Treated or processed sausages and meats have a brighter color than the real ones and the taste is not as it should be. Eggs, wine, and even fruits and vegetables, have a color and taste that is different than the natural ones. At this point, with respect to many honest producers, I must admit that not all the products we find on the market are artificially colored or flavored.

I am referring to the organic fruit and vegetable markets. Organic farming is a sector that is still underestimated, but surely it will become an agricultural model in the future. Sooner or later man will open his eyes (in part, he is already doing so) and will no longer buy products derived from chemical agriculture, namely, the traditional one. We can already notice how many companies have realized what is the right direction, and they are on the way to changing it. Those who do not comply will be excluded from the market.

In the name of our health, we must support, strengthen, and stimulate the following sectors:[53]

> the organic vegetable market;

> the organic milk market;

> the organic egg market.

THE ETERNAL DILEMMA

Someone might be asking, "If everything we eat is so contaminated, why do we live longer than before?" We have already answered this question in part when we talked about the environment in general.

Now I will try to examine this topic more deeply through its most important subclass: nutrition. Even though the idea that our great-grandparents were nourished in a healthier way than we are is widespread, since the human lifespan has gradually increased, it is believed that the current nutritional system is perfectly balanced and that very sophisticated culinary art does not have any negative influence on health. In the opinion of many people, the chemical and pharmaceutical industries have contributed substantially to the extension of life. All these controversies aside, we should perhaps look more closely at the extent to which those claims are true.

On the one hand, it is true that 150 years ago the earth, the water, and the atmosphere were not as contaminated as they are today. On the other hand, it is equally true that our great-grandparents

---

53 I specified on purpose these three sectors and I did not simply say the organic sector, because today the organic industry is also applied to many foods that are harmful to our health, such as meat, coffee, and other types of food. If a food itself is bad, it does not matter whether or not it is organic. What is the difference between a normal and an organic poison? We will talk about this later in the book.

cooked most of their food. So cooking was considered a true "predigestion," preparing food for absorption and assimilation by the organism. The more it was used, the better it was for the people.

Then there was the invention of pasteurization as a way of protecting health from pathogenic microorganisms. The process is named after the French chemist Louis Pasteur, who performed the first pasteurization together with Claude Bernard on April 20, 1862.

The terror of microorganisms as generators of disease has spread worldwide and continues even today. It was highlighted in newspapers, in books, and in gastronomy manuals that everything had to be boiled and pasteurized.

A DIFFERENT REALITY

It was only after 1900, when the Swiss nutritionist Dr. Oskar Maximilian Bircher-Benner created granola and demonstrated the enormous importance of fruits and vegetables, that a new opinion trend arose which aimed at a healthier lifestyle.

Dr. Bircher suggested that fruits, vegetables, and cereals were more nutritious than meat products. Recall that granola is a mixture of cereal flakes, dried fruit (raisins, apples, bananas), oil seeds (hazelnuts, almonds), and honey. This recipe has been developed in order to prepare a healthy and complete meal.

At the beginning of the last century it was concluded that it was necessary to undertake a healthier and more nutritious way of life. As a result, associations and institutions advocating a change of mentality were formed. Much has been published on natural cures and diets based on raw food. In this aspect, conferences and training courses organized by these companies proved to be very effective, so effective that even some doctors changed their minds.

Other factors have also contributed to increasing the life span. In addition to those already mentioned, we can list modern surgery and better care of patients. Thanks to these factors, many people have gained years of life. The pharmaceutical industry has contributed also to the prolongation of human life, keeping diseases at bay but without eradicating them.

It could be said that patients do not die but neither do they heal. Moreover, after the treatment the disease either reappears later or degenerates into other diseases. To really cure a disease you have to eliminate the cause, otherwise any kind of treatment makes no sense.

MODERN MEDICINE

The way modern medicine treats sick people can be compared to a man who finds himself in a boat that is taking on water from a hole. Instead of covering the hole where the water comes in, he fights to empty the boat using a bowl. After a while he is completely exhausted. He keeps floating a little more, but eventually drowns.

Water represents the dirtiness, the waste, and residues with which our sick bodies are continuously overloaded through poor nutrition and toxic drugs. In the end, the patient "drowns" in them. The bowl represents the way in which both medicine and modern surgery can help the situation.

One hundred years ago people did not even have the bowl to get rid of the water. This is why lifespans were shorter than today. Many people cannot believe that there is a miraculous cure known and feasible to any person of any social stratum. In reality, this cure exists. It has been tested and proven. However, it is not being spread for two reasons:

1) Most of the doctors exclude it from the very beginning. In fact, the low price of the diet in question is of little interest for them because they would gain little or even nothing from promoting it. Therefore, doctors can never truly recognize the merits of this type of diet.

2) Patients are more interested in the pleasures of the belly than in their own health. Yet they do not know that a raw-food diet can satisfy their palate as well. No one thinks that death can be hidden behind a wrong diet. Leonardo Da Vinci, the genius of the Renaissance, used to say, "Our bodies become more and more the tombs of animals."

WHAT DO WE REALLY KNOW?

Our universities almost exclusively teach chemotherapy, pharmacotherapy, and surgery. This constitutes a crime. Actually, that means a longer life without health. It is just pain, suffering, and bitterness.

We all know that there are many different types of diets. We can count at least a hundred of them. Among the best known are the vegan, the low-fat, the macrobiotic, the dissociated, the Mediterranean, and the raw-food diet.

The latter type is perhaps the least known. If I had to examine these diets one by one, I could write a whole book. So I will just tell a short story.

In 2005, I was told, with an air of triumph, that a follower of a natural diet died of cancer. She lived in Milan and was 46 years old. Hearing the sad news, I was surprised because I could not understand how such a thing was possible, so at my own expense I decided to investigate the woman in question and went to visit her relatives.

Being a researcher, for me it was important to know the real cause of her death, even more so because before this case I happened to meet people who told me of a relative or friend who died suddenly even though they had never smoked or drank alcohol. Well, not smoking or drinking is insufficient. The most important thing is nutrition.

Eventually I found out that this lady was not a follower of the raw-food diet. She was a vegetarian.[54] Many people think that there is no difference between these two diets, but they are wrong. It is true that vegetarians give up eating meat, but they cook the vast majority of their food. Even if the foods are cooked with caution,

---

54 Some people have asked me if Paavo Airola was a raw foodist. It is quite known that he recommended the use of a diet consisting of 75 percent of raw foods and 25 percent of cooked foods. So we cannot say that he was a raw foodist. He was, instead, a vegetarian. It should also be said that the raw foodists are not all equal. Although everyone eats 100 percent raw foods, some people also eat raw milk and raw eggs (as I do), whereas others do not. Another thing that needs to be said is that even if nutrition is what affects our life span the most (about 36 percent), it is only the tip of the iceberg. In fact, there are also other factors, such as the sun, the water, the air, thinking, physical activity, intoxication, and so on. Paavo Airola made some very serious mistakes too. First of all, he used food supplements (that must be absolutely avoided!) in order to integrate certain vitamins and minerals lacking in the vegetable world, such as vitamin B12 for example. He did not know that this problem could be overcome by the simple consumption of raw milk and raw eggs. I do not know if it is a coincidence, but several scientific studies (discussed in the second volume) attribute to food supplements a high risk of stroke. A stroke was exactly what caused the death of this famous nutritionist 64 years ago.

for example with steam, there is no difference between this type of cooking and others. In both cases, the most important substances, i.e., the enzymes, are destroyed.

Another worrying fact is the misuse of the word "natural." This adjective is erroneously associated with many diets such as the vegetarian and other diets. In reality, "natural" refers to very few things that are really natural, i.e., to foods that not only have to be produced in a natural way but also may not have undergone any sort of modification or treatment.

DOUBLE LIES

All those TV commercials advertising steamers, pressure cookers, or double-bottom cookers (1 cm), which say that cooking is done uniformly and that it does not destroy vitamins, make me smile. Even in this case, it does not matter if the enzymes are destroyed first on the bottom of the saucepan and then on the surface or if they are destroyed all at once uniformly, as in the case of the double boiler.

The only advantage of this last type of cookware is that the food does not stick to the bottom and it does not burn. Pressure cookers, for the sake of faster cooking, destroy and impoverish the food even more. In fact, if by traditional cooking foods lose up to 60 percent of their nutritional value, using pressure cookers we can lose even 80 percent of the nutritional value.

Not only are enzymes destroyed, but also a great part of the vitamins. One of the most important, i.e., vitamin C, whose primary role is the purification of our blood, gets totally lost through cooking.

AND STEAM

By boiling and steaming we destroy all minerals, so legumes and vegetables lose all their nutritional properties. Proteins as well lose two-thirds of their nutritional value with the cooking—one part with the coagulation, the other part with the destruction. At the same time, the now modified proteins produce more acids and residues following metabolization.

The lack of enzymes causes more than three-fourths of mineral salts, which are very important for the cells of our body, to be unassimilated by the organism; thus they are deposited as residues. With such huge losses, we are likely to be undernourished even if our stomach is full. Cooking degrades even starch and fructose, and their chemical composition changes totally. This represents a real danger for us and opens a way to obesity. These chemical changes do not exist in raw foods.

Taking into consideration another example, diabetics include in their diet dried fruit but not cooked fruit. This is a confirmation that the change which sugar and starch undergoes during cooking is harmful for our health. Fruits and vegetables should not be cooked or sterilized in any way. The only way of conservation should be through the refrigerator and drying (natural drying and at room temperature. And not in the oven, as we do today, because it would destroy their nutrients).

Fats and oils are those foods that are subject to the greatest damage. I am not referring here just to their cooking but also to their production process: for example: hot pressed oils. We will discuss in detail this topic in the chapter "Fats" in the second volume.

HERE THEY ARE . . . ARTIFICIAL REINFORCEMENTS

Cooking compromises even the aroma and flavor of food. This is why we need to create artificial supports, for example, salt and sugar. Both of them are very harmful, yet they are the most used. We will speak about this aspect later in the text.

It has been observed that individuals who eat cooked foods consume a quantity of food which is three to four times higher than those who eat raw food. This happens for two simple reasons:

1) Cooked foods, being poor from the nutritional point of view, lead us to eat more in order to get the amount of vitamins, minerals, and enzymes that our body normally needs.

2) Boiling[55] decreases the volume of food significantly. As a result, fatigue can keep under control the deposits and the increase in body mass. In addition, the expenses generated by cooking food are much higher. This is what man sacrifices for an insignificant culinary pleasure!

It is true that man has been cooking his food for thousands of years. However, man has been living on the Earth for much longer and is biologically and physiologically programmed to eat without the use of fire, just like all the other animals. Violating the rules of nature produces consequences that are easily observable: no other animals on the planet cook their own food and no other animals except humans and domesticated animals suffer from so many problems and diseases. Moreover, taste can easily be reeducated, since it is a habit.

As for the satisfaction of the palate, I like my current nutrition more than what I used to eat in the past!

---

55 And as a result, food becomes more caloric.

ZARO AĞA

Zaro Ağa (1777–June 29, 1934) was the longest-living man in Turkey. Zaro was born in Bitlis, in the Kurdistan province, during Ottoman Turkey. As a young man he worked in construction. Then he moved to Istanbul where he worked as a porter for over a hundred years and finally retired after working as a janitor. He was a great attraction for the press during the last years of his life.

During his long life he traveled to many countries, including the United States, the United Kingdom, Italy, and France.

In his 1976 book, Arthur C. Custance quotes an article in *News Review* of December 22, 1938, according to which the age of Zaro Ağa was certified at 164 years. Despite this fact, in accordance with the death certificate prepared by his doctor, Zaro Ağa had no more than 157 years. When he died, there was no debate about his actual age anyway.

Zaro Ağa survived 10 sultans and a president and lived through six wars. In 1798, under the command of Cezzar Ahmet Pasha, he fought against Napoleon's army. He also participated in the Russian-Ottoman war in 1828, where he was wounded in one leg.

He married 11 times and had 36 children. The last child, a daughter, was born when he was 96 years old.

In 1929, the Great Depression hit Turkey. At that time Zaro Ağa had become a celebrity. He participated in an advertising campaign that recommended the use of domestic products to save the country, while encouraging people to adopt new economic policies.

ZARO'S SECRET

Zaro remained physically strong until the end of his days, always joking and smiling. In an interview in 1930, while he was in the United States, he was asked the secret of his long life.

Ağa Zaro answered, "I do not drink and I do not smoke. I eat fruits, vegetables, and yogurt. I also eat raisins, nuts, olive oil, figs, and many other things."

The following is an example of one of his menus during his stay in the United States:

Breakfast: an uncooked egg, a glass of raw milk, and an orange.

Lunch: cauliflower, spinach, and a plate of vegetables.

Dinner: cheese curdled with vegetables.

Just before his death he said, "My time has come." After his death, his body was sent to the U.S. for research purposes. For years scholars have examined the heart, liver, and brain of this super-centenarian in order to discover the secret of his longevity. For some years, his brain was exhibited at the Museum of Health in Sultanahmet, Turkey. His favorite foods were bulgur (wheat sprouts) and yogurt.

DO WOMEN LIVE LONGER THAN MEN?

The next myth I want to debunk is still very controversial in the scientific world. It is the belief that women naturally live longer than men. There is nothing further from the truth than this statement.[56] Everything in nature is balanced and in perfect harmony. Why would the Creator have given more days to women? Believing this statement is like believing that the heart is naturally more durable than our lungs. What would be the sense of the existence of the heart without lungs? Aren't they complementary? If the heart stops beating, the lungs die, and vice versa.

To ensure the survival and continuity of our species, man and woman need each other equally. This fundamental principle of survival has been imprinted into the DNA of all living beings since the dawning of all creation.

---

56 This is good news either for men or for women, because a wife has not been programmed to live her last years of life without a husband.

For a long time doctors have believed, or have wanted us to believe, that the greater longevity of women was due to estrogen, the main female sex hormone. This theory was put forward by pharmaceutical companies with the aim of creating a more lucrative market for their synthetic hormones given to women in menopause.

It is typical of pharmaceutical companies to dramatically amplify and exaggerate the importance of any substance in our organism, substances they can imitate artificially and proclaim as the solution.

Still today, estrogen deficiency is proclaimed loudly by doctors, pharmaceutical advertising, and many industry publications. It is thought to be the primary cause of all the symptoms attributed to menopause and post-menopause, such as mood swings, depression, vaginal dryness, loss of libido, cardiovascular disease, and osteoporosis acceleration.

But is there really something like a lack of estrogen? While it is true that menopause is associated with decreased levels of estrogen, it is not true that this phenomenon causes all the symptoms of menopause.

In 1991 the Women's Health Initiative (WHI) was launched. It was the largest research program aimed at addressing the most common causes of death, disability, and poor quality of life for women after menopause, including cardiovascular disease, cancer, and osteoporosis. The study lasted 15 years and involved 191,808 postmenopausal women who were, at least initially, healthy.

These clinical studies were developed to test the effects of postmenopausal hormone therapy, of the modification of diet, and of calcium and vitamin D in heart disease, fractures, cancer, breast cancer, and colorectal cancer. The results were surprising.

The study revealed that estrogen and progestin hormone therapy after menopause not only did not protect women from heart disease, as doctors had previously thought, but actually increased their risk of heart attack, stroke, and breast cancer. The risk of breast cancer was twice as high in women following hormonal therapy.

Another interesting aspect is that scientists have found no significant link between the use of multivitamins and a reduced risk of developing cancer or cardiovascular disease, or even death. In other words, post-menopausal women who took multivitamins or integrators seemed to have the same risk of developing the most common types of cancer or cardiovascular disease as women who did not take multivitamin supplements.

Furthermore, the Women's Health Initiative showed that hormone therapy in women aged 65 years or older may increase the likelihood of having difficulty with thinking skills and memory. It increases the risk of dementia and cognitive impairment. In addition, women who have undergone this therapy showed a higher rate of stroke and brain injury than those who had not followed it. Many other studies have led to similar conclusions.

Finally, the last little-known aspect of hormone replacement therapy (HRT) is that it is about addictive drugs. It is very likely that the widespread prescription of synthetic hormones to women will be remembered as the biggest mess in medical history.

It is true that women have a higher life expectancy than men and that their average lifespan is about five-to-six years longer. There are also countries where this difference reaches 15 to 20 years, such as Russia.

If we calculate the global age average, we can notice that women live almost 12 years longer than men. About this subject, there are a lot of speculations and opinions ranging from estrogen to genes. In fact, the truth is quite different and is kept well hidden.

There are two factors that affect the longevity of women. The first factor is that women are more concerned about their health. They are more likely to go to the doctor regularly. They follow carefully a certain diet, are more careful about their appearance and, in general, do everything to keep young as long as possible. Men, on the other hand, lead an irregular lifestyle, drink more alcohol, smoke more, eat more fatty foods, often snack while they are in a hurry, and spend less time doing physical exercise.

The second factor is that men take more risks than women. If we look at death statistics, both at work and in leisure time, we can see that death statistics for men exceed the statistics for women. These data affect the general statistics of life expectancy.

Even among depressed people, the mortality rate is higher in men when compared to women. This is because their suicide attempts are more "successful" than women's.

It isn't possible to maintain that women are biologically predisposed to live longer than men. Instead, it would be better to say that women are more balanced, prudent, and calm.

A German study, conducted at the University of Surrey, shows that married men live longer in comparison to single men. In fact, encouraged by their wives, husbands eat more healthfully, have medical checkups more often, and devote more time to physical exercise.

CHAPTER 7

THE SECRETS OF WATER

> Water is the primordial element of life, regeneration and purity.
>
> Thales of Miletus

Water is an important nutrient for our bodies. It is so important that, in its absence, death will occur within a few days. About 70 percent of the human body consists of water, which must be continually replenished because every day we lose at least half a liter just through breathing and perspiration.

Water is necessary for digestion and for waste elimination. It works as a lubricant of joints and eyes and is essential for the regulation of body temperature.

Either drinks or food will supply our organism with water. The daily need for an adult is about 2.5 liters. Of these 2.5 liters, about 300 ml derive from the reactions that occur in the body while the rest must come from nutrition in the form of beverages and foods such as fruits and vegetables. When we make a physical effort or when the weather is particularly hot, we should drink more than usual to compensate for the water lost through rapid breathing and sweating. Eliminating a lot of water through sweating also means losing a lot of mineral salts, which should be readily replenished through fruits and vegetables[57] in order to avoid serious damage to our organism.

Drinking plenty of water can also dilute and eliminate waste quickly through the urine. Those who drink little water may suffer from headaches, difficulty in concentrating, constipation, and other ailments.

Water is an essential commodity for life. And it is a renewable resource on our planet. Every living entity is linked to water, and all human activities are bound to access to water.

THERE IS LESS WATER THAN YOU THINK

The first impression that our planet gives to a child when he looks at it for the first time in a world atlas is that the Earth is literally under water.

Actually, 71 percent of our planet is covered by water, namely, about two-thirds. This is the reason for the idea that there is plenty of water, imprinted in our subconscious since we were children.

However, things are not always as they seem. First of all, it should be said that of the approximately 1,400 million km³ of water covering the Earth, 97.5 percent is made up of salt water (seas and oceans). That water cannot be used for the usual human purposes

---

57 Mineral salts have to be reintegrated through fruits and vegetables and not through water or food integrators, as many people think. This will be explained later in the chapter.

without facing very high economic and ecological costs. The rest of the water, about 2.5 percent, is fresh water and can be used by man. Fresh water can be found in glaciers and perpetual snow, in the ground, in rivers and lakes.

Of all the 2.5 percent of fresh water, what is directly available for the needs of man is constituted by the water surface of lakes and rivers, and partially by underground water, equal to approximately 0.03 percent; in other words, three parts out of 10,000. This is just a small fraction compared to the amount of water on Earth.

With a simple arithmetic calculation (1,400/10,000 × 3) we can see that fresh water directly available for human needs is about 0.42 million km^3. If all the water on Earth was equivalent to 100 liters, fresh water that can be used for drinking would amount to about 30 ml, i.e., the equivalent of two tablespoons.

WATER POLLUTION

The increase of world population implies a growing demand for water. But at the same time, pollution blocks the access to important supply sources. It is believed that water, either due to its shortage or to its poor quality, is related to approximately 80 percent of all the world's diseases and about 30 percent of deaths.

Today, compared to a hundred years ago, the situation has changed. The world population has more than tripled and the number of industries has soared. Factories produce huge amounts of artificial chemicals that are hardly degradable (plastics, nylon, detergents) and which contain in some cases very toxic metals such as mercury, nickel, zinc, and chromium. The domestic sewage and rubbish of our daily lives, like detergents, solvents, and dyes, end up in the waters of rivers, lakes, and seas. All these poisons contain such a quantity of synthetic and organic matter that the naturally potential self-purification of water is blocked.

Furthermore, the pollution caused by these substances has harmful effects on marine organisms and the animals that eat them. Humans and birds are poisoned as well. The problem with water, in fact, is much more complex than it seems to be.

THE WAYS OF POLLUTION ARE ENDLESS

In addition to the spills poured out directly into the rivers or the sea, part of the pollution comes through precipitation.[58]

Agriculture also plays a role in contaminating groundwater, watercourses, and the sea, because every year huge amounts of residues of chemical fertilizers, insecticides, and pesticides reach them.

Another way of pollution affecting marine waters is due to the oil that gets to the sea by different causes: loss from the pipes of the coastal refineries, accidents involving large tankers, and improper washing of the oil tankers in open sea. Unfortunately, the list of the forms of pollution does not end here. Describing all the damage that man is causing to our hydrosphere would take floods of ink.

It is said that water is a renewable element, yet its renewal takes several years. For the oceans and ice caps it takes around 4,000 years, and for the deep deposits about 10,000 years. Therefore, water is a renewable element but it is limited. Furthermore, its capacity

---

58 When water vapor in the seas and oceans mixes with the polluted atmosphere, rain, snow, fog, and acid dew are formed. This type of precipitation is devastating for the flora and the environment.

for renewal can be quickly altered if we withdraw large amounts of ground water, especially if we consider that these deposits were formed over many thousands of years and are now consumed at the rate of a million cubic meters per year.

A COLOSSAL DEAL

It is estimated that from 1950 to 2000, water per capita availability has fallen by an average of 16,800 cubic meters to 6,800, and in 2020 the number of people who will not have access to water will reach four billion, that is, half the world's population.

At this point, we have to clarify that the availability of water resources and access to water are not the same thing. Neither are they linked by a cause-and-effect relationship. Some countries with limited water availability are the leading places in water usage. For example, in the U.S., California has a per capita consumption of 4,100 liters per day in spite of not having a large supply. On the contrary, in Brazil water abounds but the majority of the population has little or no access to drinking water.

It seems incredible, but some people are even happy with this emergency and take advantage of the situation. For many multinational companies, as well as governments, water is in fact primarily a commodity, an asset that will become—because of its limited availability—the deal of the twenty-first century, i.e., the blue gold.

Governments and municipalities are opening the door to massive intervention of privatization of water. We can include here many multinationals too, starting with the giants of mineral water that buy sources and springs around the world and invest in so-called "purified water" (water with added minerals).

People suffering from diseases caused by water occupy more than half of the world's hospital beds, and 6,000 children die every day from drinking polluted water.

The United Nations predicts that by 2025 two-thirds of the world's population will live in regions with a shortage of water resources.

WATER CLASSIFICATION

Based on the source and type of treatment, drinking water can be classified into five groups:

1. spring water;
2. well water (artesian and ground water);
3. purified water (reverse osmosis or other methods);
4. mineral water (bottled);
5. tap water (lakes and rivers).

TAP WATER

We all know that most of the water that comes to our houses comes from lakes and rivers. Now it is also possible to know its characteristics.

Although filtered well and regularly controlled polluting substances, like fertilizers, pesticides, industrial chemicals, and heavy metals such as cadmium, lead, aluminum, and other poisonous substances may be present in the water.

To overcome this problem, many people have started to drink

bottled water. Even though people drink mineral water, when they cook everybody uses water from the tap. In this way they are not giving any importance (or they are underestimating it) to the water quality with which foods are prepared.

This happens because it is widely believed that the water that is not good to drink is good for cooking since boiling will improve its quality. This belief is totally wrong.

None of the harmful substances listed above can become good by boiling, nor can they be eliminated. On the contrary, because of the evaporation effect, the substances in question are gathered together and are even more absorbed in the foods during cooking. There are not two types of water, one to drink and the other one with which to cook. There is only one type: the water for food use.

Furthermore, in order to disinfect water from microorganisms, chlorine—which is another poison—is added to tap water. Many scientific studies have shown that there is a correlation between the ingestion of chlorinated water and the occurrence of some types of cancer (bladder, rectum) and other potential risks for human health, such as spontaneous abortions and malformations of newborns.

Would anyone put two drops of bleach in the water then give it to their child to drink to make it safer? I don't think so. Nevertheless, it is what we do when we add chlorine (sodium hypochlorite) to water to kill viruses and bacteria. After all, where do the bodies of these poisoned microorganisms end up? Can this water really be defined as drinking water?

But this is not the end of the story. Aluminum sulfate is often added to the water during the purification process to eliminate the particles in suspension. It is then removed by filtration. However, a certain amount of particles still manage to pass through the filter.

A SOURCE OF DISEASES

It is no longer a secret that we live better and longer in areas where so-called civilization has not been established yet, despite the improved hygienic conditions of life and the undeniable scientific progress of medicine and surgery.

In 1989, an article that appeared in the medical journal *The Lancet*[59] pointed out that in areas where the amount of aluminum in drinking water is greater than 0.11 mg/liter there is an increased risk of Alzheimer's disease compared to those areas in which such concentration is less than 0.01 mg/liter.

In the waters of some rivers and lakes from which drinking water is drawn, chemicals similar to estrogen, hormones used in contraceptive pills were discovered. These substances have been linked to reduced male fertility in fish and reptiles present in these waters. Some researchers, together with some environmental organizations, are increasingly concerned that they may also have an effect on human fertility.

Also, due to the passage of water through pipes, lead is dissolved from the walls into small particles which, when ingested together with water, not only can cause poor coordination but can also block children's growth and damage their nervous systems, kidneys, and reproductive organs.

---

59 Martyn, C. N., et al., "Geographical Relation Between Alzheimer's Disease and Aluminum in Drinking Water," *The Lancet*, Vol. 333, 8629, 14 Jan. 1989., pp. 61–62.

NITRATES AND WATER

Nitrate is an inorganic compound that is found more frequently in ground water in rural areas. It is composed of one atom of nitrogen (N) and three atoms of oxygen (O). Its chemical symbol is NO_3.

Nitrate itself is not so noxious, but under particular conditions (heat, bacteria, long preservation) it can be transformed into nitrite, i.e., to NO_2, which is very toxic for man.

At this point, it is not difficult to imagine that inside our body nitrates find the ideal conditions for turning into nitrites. In fact, apart from the body heat, inside the human organism there are proper bacteria that transform the nitrates into nitrites.

The formation of nitrates is mainly due to fertilizers, septic and storage systems, or the spreading of fertilizers. The nitrogen contained in fertilizers that are not absorbed by plants ends up in groundwater in the form of nitrate.

The water with nitrates and processed foods with nitrates should therefore be avoided or, at least, should not be heated. In fact, worldwide associations for cancer research invite us not to use water containing nitrates either for drinking or for cooking.

The excessive use of nitrates and nitrites is also responsible for the increase in the incidence of diseases such as diabetes, Parkinson's disease, and Alzheimer's. This was revealed in an epidemiological study of the Rhode Island Hospital and Brown University, published in the *Journal of Alzheimer's Disease*.

When nitrates reach the stomach and are transformed into nitrites, they can react with the amines contained in foods to form nitrosamines. Nitrosamines are carcinogens, substances related to some forms of gastric cancer.

Moreover, in children, nitrates can cause a particularly serious anemia. When nitrate is transformed into nitrite in the stomach of a child, it also reacts with hemoglobin, limiting the ability of the latter to deliver oxygen in the blood and then its flow to the brain. Some scientific studies have also shown that regular consumption of water with more than 10 mg/liter by pregnant women can cause miscarriages.

By boiling water at 100° C, double nitrates in a few minutes because of the amount of evaporation. So, water with 35/40 mg/liter, even though being "according to the law" for some countries, when boiled reaches 70/80 mg and thus becomes "non-according to the law."

We must choose water whose nitrate concentration is less than 3 mg/liter or, even better, totally devoid of nitrates. We should be wary of mineral waters that do not report on the label the amount of nitrates because usually manufacturers hide very high nitrate values.

NITRATES AND VEGETABLES

Nitrates are also absorbed through vegetables fertilized with nitrogen-based preparations. Plants, in fact, use nitrates to synthesize the key elements for their growth with the help of sunlight. The greater the exposure of plants to sunlight, the lower their content of nitrates. Therefore, the vegetables grown in open fields contain fewer nitrates than those produced in a greenhouse. Summer vegetables contain fewer nitrates than winter crops. And vegetables collected after sunset, contain fewer nitrates than those collected in the morning.

Some time ago a friend told me, "Nowadays it is useless to eat fresh fruits and raw vegetables because they are full of nitrates."

I must say that this statement is true, but only in part. It is true that vegetables are the main source of nitrates if they are fertilized with chemical fertilizers, but on the other hand they also contain a number of essential micronutrients and antioxidants that inhibit the formation of N-nitroso compounds.

If vegetables are cooked then, yes, it is true that they can no longer protect us from all the toxins used by the agriculture industry because cooking destroys all or part of their natural defenses such as enzymes, antioxidants, vitamins, and other toxic inhibitors.

We gain more benefit by eating fresh fruits and raw vegetables chemically treated than cooking them or not eating them at all. Ideally, we should eat only fruits and vegetables organically grown.

An Italian study on the correlation between dietary factors and cancer, conducted in different regions of the world characterized by either a low risk of developing the disease or a high one, highlighted an inversely proportional relationship between cancer incidence and the consumption of fresh fruits and raw vegetables. The study, which lasted five years, revealed that in areas where fruits and vegetables were not consumed regularly, there was a higher incidence of cancer as compared to those areas where fruits and vegetables were contaminated; despite this fact they were regularly consumed.

THE HARDER THE WATER THE MORE IT KILLS

Louis Pasteur said, "90 percent of diseases come from water." And the French hydrologist Louis-Claude Vincent added, "Tuberculosis, cancer, and all degenerative diseases come from the uncontrolled use of drinking water."

Unfortunately, these heavy allegations have never been given due consideration because the serious health consequences due to unhealthy water do not appear immediately, but in the medium and long term.

In a statistical work many years ago, Professor Vincent clearly demonstrated the existence of a relationship between the quality of drinking water of a given population and the mortality rate.

Vincent conducted the research when he was still working as an advisor for the French Government. He had at his disposal all the statistics on disease incidence and mortality rates in France, as well as in Europe and the United States.

The study clearly showed that where drinking water was purer, the mortality rate was also lower. In areas with a high mortality rate the water was hard, chemically treated, and chlorinated. At the same time, surface waters were chemically contaminated by industry and agriculture. Therefore, hard water, contaminated, treated, and chlorinated, is directly related to a high mortality rate.

SPRING WATER—LIVING WATER

Spring water is the best water. It comes out from the Earth's surface in a natural way, without altering the delicate water balance of the aquifer that nourishes it. Spring waters, of course, surface; i.e., they are not artificially extracted from the ground.

For those who have the opportunity to drink it, pristine spring water is the best choice. These springs must be far away from residential areas, landfills, factories, and everything else that may somehow contaminate its aquifers. It can be found in the mountains, in the forests, and in the hills.

Needless to say, the best springs are those that are in the mountains. However, those present in the forests and hills are also valid if they are not polluted.

In villages and in the countryside, for example, farmers already know which are the sources of good water. With the word "good" we mean that the water is "light," namely, with less salt and a delicate flavor. Practically, it is tasteless. An expert in water can recognize this type of spring. Once the spring is found, what remains is to tap into it.

In the legends of many peoples, the water of some springs was even called living water for the miraculous effect it had on health. It was said that people who drank the living water from those springs were healed from all disease. Moreover, they remained younger.

For a better understanding of the value that many people attributed to the springs, it is sufficient to read their ancient mythologies. Many of them tell us, for example, that heroes who died were given the water to drink to turn them back to life. Of course, these are just legends, but we cannot deny the fact that they hide a little bit of truth. It is not a coincidence that 80 percent of long-living persons always drink spring water.

WELLS

Generally, the word "well" indicates an artificial structure. It usually has a circular shape and varies greatly in size. From a well we can normally extract water from underground aquifers. These may be groundwater aquifers or artesian aquifers, depending on whether the flow of water that permeates them is "free surface" or "under pressure."

THE WATER-TABLE WELL

In common slang, a water-table well is the classic well that is often found in the courtyards of countryside houses or in the cloisters of monasteries It is of a large diameter and is covered with brick or stone Also, the wells of large diameter with rings made of concrete,[60] which can be considered the modern version of the old well, are normally called water-table wells. These wells are usually not more than 10–20 meters deep and, therefore, they are mainly used to capture the water of superficial aquifers.

Water-table wells have the advantage of carrying out the functions of well and storage tank simultaneously. This is why they are also called well-tanks. In many villages of the Third World today, this type of well is still the only source of drinking water, as well as the only source of water used for irrigation and rearing livestock.

These wells are also used or can be used in industrialized countries, especially in houses with adjoining vegetable gardens and an orchard for family use where the water supplied from the public aqueduct is often not enough to meet all needs.

Also, it should be pointed out that, because of pollution, many groundwater aquifers have been contaminated and consequently the water-table wells are too. Therefore, today most of the water that comes from these aquifers is no longer considered safe drinking water.

In general, water-table wells can be used only for non-potable domestic uses or for irrigation purposes.

---

60 The best water-table wells remain those of the past, namely, those constructed with rocks. I do not recommend modern wells because in the construction of their prefabricated rings, chemical solvents are used. They are not ideal for potable use.

THE ARTESIAN WELL

The artesian well is a deeply-drilled well through which the water is forced upward under pressure, consequently creating the static level of the well.

This type of well owns the origin of its name to the Count of Artois in France, where the first well with the canonical features of an artesian well was dug in 1126.

It is obvious, therefore, that artesian water is much cleaner than groundwater. In fact, being extracted from the depths of the Earth, the artesian water is protected by various layers of clay and rock.

Moreover, the artesian well has no openings toward the Earth's surface and, therefore, the water never comes into contact with air. In this way it is protected against atmospheric pollution and any other type of contamination.

There are numerous benefits that can be obtained from an artesian well. For example, we can mention its use in homes where there is no water supply, for the irrigation of gardens and orchards, and for agricultural and industrial irrigation. Having an artesian well at home is like having a private source of mineral water.

MINERAL WATER

We consider natural mineral waters those waters which, having an origin from an underground aquifer or from a subterranean reservoir, come from one or more natural springs or perforated sources and have special hygienic characteristics and properties favorable to health.

Worldwide, there are over 3,000 brands of mineral water

commercially available. However, in many places the term "mineral water" is often used to refer to sparkling water in order to distinguish it from tap water.

According to their origin, true mineral waters are divided into spring water and artesian water. Bottled water is of either type. It seems incredible, but only 20 percent of mineral waters available for sale are of a spring nature. In any case, both artesian and spring water would be excellent water if it were not for certain drawbacks:

1. the plastic in which they are bottled;
2. the cost (up to 10,000 times more expensive than tap water);
3. transport;
4. incomplete information on labels;
5. the depletion of groundwater aquifers.

THE PLASTIC

The mineral water container is made of polyethylene terephthalate (PET). The PET is part of the polyester family and is obtained with terephthalic acid and ethylene glycol, both derivatives of crude oil.

The most authoritative observatory on environment trends of the planet, the Worldwatch Institute, in its annual State of the World 2004, in the chapter "Bottled water" by Paul McRandle, states, "The production of one kilogram of PET requires 17.5 kg of water and releases 40 grams of hydrocarbons, 25 grams of sulfur oxides, 18 grams of carbon monoxide, and 2.3 kg of carbon dioxide."

Since a PET bottle of 1.5 liters weighs about 35 grams, with a kilo of PET you can produce about 30 bottles. Therefore, carrying 45 liters of water consumes almost half of them.

Researchers from Worldwatch do not mince words in denouncing such an obvious issue and at the same time the more forgotten issue of this opulent time, "Consumers are not powerless spectators. Ultimately, they are choosing what to buy. So they are the ones who can begin a change."

A report by the Earth Policy Institute in Washington, D.C., estimated that in 2004, the global consumption of bottled water reached 154 billion liters. These figures correspond to an increased demand of 57 percent compared to the 98 billion liters that were consumed five years earlier. Only in the U.S., to produce plastic bottles more than 17 million barrels of oil were used. This is enough to fuel more than one million cars in the United States for a year. At a global level, about 2.7 million tons of plastic per year are used to bottle the water.

It is therefore evident that the demand for bottled water is increasing the production of waste and the consumption of large amounts of energy. We can drink a bottle of water in just two minutes, but to decompose a plastic bottle takes up to 1,000 years.

WHERE DOES THE PLASTIC END UP?

Only a small portion of the plastic bottles are recovered or end up in landfills. The majority are lost in the seas, oceans, forests, and fields.

According to several studies, plastics account for about 70–80 percent of the macroscopic marine debris. Just as an example, at the center of the Pacific Ocean there is a mass of plastic waste twice the size of Texas. It is called the Pacific Trash Vortex. And this is not an isolated case. In the seas and oceans all over the world there are thousands of "plastic islands."

This fact does not constitute a harmless presence. As a matter of fact, in the world there could be at least 267 species, including sea turtles, seabirds, and marine mammals, in whose stomachs large or small pieces of plastic are found.

Another problem is that the majority of people neglect the potential impact of plastics on our health. In fact, unknown and hidden information for many people is that plastics release potentially toxic substances into the water we drink. Numerous scientific investigations have shown the harmfulness not only of plastic bottles (PET) but also of any kind of food and industrial plastic containers.

HOW MUCH DOES IT COST US?

The government concession tax on a company that extracts and bottles water costs on average €3,000 per year. A company extracts and bottles about 100 million liters a year on average. This means that against a paltry concession, companies extract from the ground 100 million liters of water per year. In fact, if we divide the amount of the tax (€3,000) by 100,000,000 liters, we can see that the cost of a liter of water[61] is only €0.00003 and a bottle of water of 1.5 liter costs €0.000045.

The total cost of a plastic bottle, i.e., the container, the cap and the label, is approximately €0.12. Even in this case, if we do the math, we see that the container costs on average 4,000 times more than the actual cost of the water.

So in the end, the price we pay for the purchase of mineral

---

61 For simplicity, I did not mention here the other costs, such as machinery, labor, etc., that have a minimal impact on the price of the mineral water.

water goes almost entirely to cover the cost of packaging, transport, and advertising. In reality, the cost to producers of the water contained in a single bottle is less than the glue on the label.

TRANSPORTATION

French mineral waters end up in the United States and American waters end up in France. A very clever way of doing things, isn't it? We are devastating the world. We are destroying each other without realizing it.

The transportation of bottled water over long distances involves the consumption of large amounts of fossil fuels. Almost a quarter of all bottled water that reaches consumers crosses national boundaries.

Ships, trains, and trucks transport the water. In 2004 for example, Nord Water, a Finnish company, bottled and shipped 1.4 million bottles of water to Saudi Arabia. This means 4,300 km away from its bottling plant in Helsinki. Mineral water is therefore transported thousands of miles from one end of the world to the other.

In order to carry 15 tons, which corresponds to 10,000 1.5 liter bottles of water, a fully functional truck consumes one liter of oil every 4 km (25 liters per 100 km). Assuming an average distance of 1,000 km, round trip, fuel consumption amounts to 250 liters, or, in other words, to 250,000 cm^3, which divided by 10,000 bottles, corresponds to 25 cm^3 of diesel per bottle.

Multiplying 25 cm^3 by 240 bottles, we can find out that the per-capita daily consumption of one liter of bottled water involves a consumption of six liters of diesel per year. To these six liters of diesel we must add the following costs:

1. The consumption of oil needed to produce plastic bottles (8.4 kg per 240 bottles).
2. The fuel consumption of trucks carrying empty bottles of plastic from the factory where they are produced to the company that bottles the water, and that of the garbage trucks that transport the containers to disposal plants.
3. The specific fuel consumption of the buyers on the way: home-supermarket-home.

LABEL INFORMATION

Many suppliers of mineral water conceal the truth about their products behind images of pure fantasy. Notice how bottled water tries to seduce us with images of mountain springs or of pristine nature. In many ways, bottled water is less regulated than tap water and, what is more, it costs from 2,000 up to 10,000 times more than tap water.

Imagine paying for anything else 2,000 times more than its real value. For example, imagine paying €4,000 for 1 kg of apples or €20,000 for 1 kg of honey.

We should also bear in mind that the term "mineral water" is used differently from country to country. For example, in the European Community, mineral water is considered only that water which originates from a groundwater aquifer or from a subterranean reservoir, comes from one or more natural or perforated springs, and which has special hygienic characteristics and properties favorable to health. In many other countries of the world, the tap water that is filtered, mineralized (addition of mineral salts) and then bottled is also considered mineral water.

Actually, one third of the mineral waters in the world come from the tap. However, as already mentioned, they still make us pay for it at a thousand times more than tap water. As we can see, the images of pristine nature in one-third of the cases are misleading.

Nevertheless, even many true mineral waters are not perfect. Another problem with mineral water, apart from the plastic, the cost, and the transportation problem, is the incomplete information on labels about the chemicals dissolved in the water. And last but not least there is the problem of the depletion of groundwater aquifers—with enormous environmental inconveniences—caused by the continuous and forced extraction of tens of millions of liters per day.

The labels, which should indicate to consumers all the biochemical characteristics of the water, are really insufficient. The water suppliers list just a very small part of the totality of the water's biochemical characteristics: some mineral salts, fixed residue, conductivity, and so on.

GUIDELINE VALUES

It is unnecessary to include in this book a detailed table on the maximum values of contaminants allowed in the water for three reasons:

1. Labels do not specify all the biochemical characteristics of the water. Therefore, it is useless to know how to read them when they do not actually report everything.

2. Reports are easily available on many government websites. Here are some examples:

✓ The United States Environmental Protection Agency (EPA);

✓ The Food and Drug Administration (FDA);

✓ The World Health Organization (WHO);

✓ The European Food Safety Authority (EFSA).

3. The more difficult a theory becomes, the more we hinder its implementation. For example, on the EPA website, within the guide *Water on tap: what you need to know*,[62] among mineral salts, disinfectants, insecticides and pesticides, which usually can be found in the water and that according to the law should not exceed a certain value, we find more than 85 contaminants. It would be a nightmare to check the presence of all these substances every time.

Moreover, even if mineral-water bottlers reported on the label all the biochemical characteristics, they would very often hide the truth. This fact has already been proved more than once by consumer associations of many countries that have begun to make several analyses of many mineral waters, finding in reality much higher values than those set by the limits. Some of this research is well known today.

For all mineral waters (for tap water as well), there are upper limits of contaminants established by the organizations mentioned above. For example, if just one contaminant exceeds its maximum value, the water in question cannot be sold.

Many offenses are due to poor preservation. I am talking about the classic bottles kept in the sunlight. As a matter of fact, bottled water can remain in circulation up to 18 months, but sometimes it is not stored in optimal conditions. Who can guarantee that the

---

62 http://water.epa.gov/drink/guide

THE SECRETS OF WATER

container and the water itself retain their chemical structure months after being bottled and in the conditions the law established?

THE SOLUTION

There is a solution, and it is even easier than we might think. Given that not everyone has access to a natural spring or artesian well, the only possibility left, but also the safest and perhaps even the best one considering the times we live in, is water purified with a reverse osmosis system.

Before analyzing this system, I would like to introduce a few guidelines for those who still drink bottled water, maybe because they do not have this purification system in their home or because they have to go out of their town or even to another country for business.

Before we get lost in formulas or chemical names listed on the bottles of mineral water, we should look at the fixed residue. It is one of the most important elements in choosing the water because it determines the lightness of mineral water. In particular, the fixed residue is the amount of inorganic substances present in the water and is normally expressed in milligrams per liter. It is obtained by evaporating the water at 100° C, and subsequently dried at 180°C.

According to the value obtained, waters are afterwards classified into:

Waters Classification	Fixed Residue
Minimally mineralized water	Less than 50 mg/L
Mineral water	Between 50 and 500 mg/L
Medium mineral water	Between 501 and 1500 mg/L
Water reach in mineral salts	Greater than 1500 mg/L

So which type of water is it better to choose among, those with great, medium, or low concentrations of mineral salts? The answer is always the one with the lowest concentrations of minerals, either for children or for adults, for healthy people or for sick ones. The lighter the water, the better it is for our health. The lower the fixed residue, the better the quality of the water.

Why this choice? Because human cells cannot assimilate all inorganic minerals and consequently they are deposited within the body resulting in functional disorders in the medium and long term.

Inorganic minerals are those that come directly from the ground and which are collected from the water that comes out of the rocks. The organic minerals, instead, are those that have already been metabolized by the plants.

The inorganic minerals present in the soil and in the water, therefore, cannot be directly metabolized by human cells; namely, they cannot be transformed into substances of the organism. They must first be metabolized by the plant cells and transformed into organic minerals. This is precisely the striking difference between water mineral salts and plant mineral salts.

It is not the same to take calcium through the water or through vegetables. The second type of calcium is organically bound; the first one is not. The second type is alive, while the first one is dead. At this point, we can generalize that all mineral salts of water are tiny pebbles which end up blocking, contaminating, and soiling our organism. In fact, it will have to work harder to get rid of them.

PAY ATTENTION TO PEBBLES

Everything has a limit, and so do our bodies. The body can expel only a very small part of these salts (stones) while the rest are buried in the dumping of our body, namely, in fats.

Here is another reason why we gain weight: the pebbles clog all filters of our organism from the kidneys to the smallest cell.

What happens when a dishwasher, washing machine, or toilet clog? The water no longer flows. The same happens in our bodies. Our cells struggle either to get the nutrients we need or to release waste products. They have difficulty even to breathe. For this reason, sick people have shortness of breath and need the oxygen tank.

A low fixed residue promotes hydration and the liquid replacement for metabolism. In addition, it dissolves the stones, increases diuresis and facilitates the elimination of toxins, uric acid, and waste products of metabolism.

A high value leads to heart failure, liver cirrhosis, kidney failure, and many other ailments. This is why we should drink only water with a fixed residue of less than 30 mg/L. Remember, the lower its value, the better.

A LOGICAL PROBLEM

Two people drink two different types of waters. The first person usually drinks water containing a fixed residue of 800 mg/L. The second one drinks water with a fixed residue of 20 mg/L. Unbeknownst to them, both types of water contain the same amount of a toxic contaminant, i.e., arsenic, which exceeds the maximum value equal to 0.01 mg/L set by the EPA and the WHO.

The two types of water contain a quantity of arsenic five times higher than that allowed by law, i.e., of 0.05 mg/L. Who is most at risk, and why?

The first person, of course. A clean body, compared to a clogged one, would take no effort to immediately eliminate the intruder because it will not be occupied or busy in the expulsion of other toxins. As a consequence, all its strengths can focus only on the toxin.

OTHER RECOMMENDATIONS

The pH is a parameter that measures the acidity of the water. We have already met it in the chapter "Acids in the Human Organism." What applies to any other solution is also valid in the case of water: if the value is equal to 7.0, the water is neutral. The more the value falls below 7.0, the more the water is acidic; the more it increases above 7.0, the more the water is alkaline. Pure water has a pH of 7.0.

Be careful: do not confuse pure water (without mineral salts), which has a pH of 7.0, with impure water which may also have a pH of 7.0 because of acid and base minerals contained in it.

Please note that the pH value of 7.0 of pure water corresponds to the internal environment of the human cell (cytoplasm) too. In fact, the pH of the human cytoplasm varies between 7.0 and 7.4, and is usually higher in cells that are growing. Furthermore, the pH of the extracellular fluids is 7.4. At this point, it is clear that ideal water should have a pH between these two values, namely, between 7.0 and 7.4.

Therefore, if we have to choose between three types of waters that have the same fixed residue of 23 mg/L, but a pH, respectively, of 6.5, 7.3 and 7.8, then we have to choose the one with the pH closer to the value mentioned above. In this case, we will opt for the water which has a pH of 7.3.

Conversely, if we have to choose between two types of water that have both a pH of 7.1, but the one has a fixed residue equal to 14 mg/L and the other equal to 28 mg/L, it is obvious that for the same pH we will choose the one with fewer mineral salts.

In any case, do not exceed the range between 6.5 and 8. All waters that have a pH less than 6.5 are too acidic, whereas those with a pH above 8 are too basic.

In comparison with food, water takes a few seconds to enter the circulation in our organism. This is why the value of its pH must be as close as possible to the values of our body.

We must also know that all kinds of sparkling waters, i.e., those containing carbon dioxide in addition, should be avoided because their acidity is too high.

Nitrates and Nitrites: We talked extensively about them in this chapter. So all I have to do is summarize. According to my experience, the optimal value not to be exceeded is 3 mg/L for nitrates and 0.005 mg/L for nitrites. If nitrites are absent, it is even better.

Hardness: It represents the value of the limestone dissolved in water expressed in "French degrees." It gives us an estimate of the presence of calcium and magnesium. The higher this value is, the more the water is considered hard. It is originated from limestone and marlstone underground.

Electrical Conductivity: This is a countercheck of the fixed residue. In fact, the greater the amount of minerals, the more the water allows the passage of electricity. It is expressed in micro Siemens per cm (μ S/cm). A greater quantity of electrolytes means a high concentration of minerals. Low values are typical of waters which are poor in salts. It is better to choose waters with values of less than 50 μ S/cm.

Other Substances: With regard to all other substances, read the section of this chapter called "The Guideline Values." The only thing I would add to what is already said is to invite readers to comply with the guide values of the above-mentioned organization, but to always choose the lowest possible value. For example, if for a pollutant or contaminant the EPA recommends not exceeding the value of 20 mg/L, we should take a good one-tenth of that value, in this case 2 mg/L.

REVERSE OSMOSIS

If we do not have a natural spring or an artesian well, the only alternative is the purification of tap water, the water-table well, or the artesian[63] well with the reverse osmosis system.

The fathers of natural medicine considered our bodies a river that harbors life and thus must be kept clean. When looking for pure water, we will have to bear in mind that the fewer elements it contains, the better its quality.

Reverse osmosis is a system that, by means of network pressure, forces the water to pass through a semipermeable membrane, which, depending on the model, retains from 95 to 99 percent of all substances contained in the water. What does this mean?

It means that everything—bacteria, viruses, pesticides, poisons, chemicals, or minerals—will be eliminated up to 99 percent. This is only the average, because for some substances, and for all bacteria and viruses, microfiltration reaches 100 percent. To give a comparison, the size of a bacterium compared to the diameter of these micropores would be like a football field that tries to pass through the eye of a needle.

At the beginning, these microfilters were designed for the military, for personal survival of the soldiers.

Theoretically, this system could also filter your urine so that you could then drink it like spring water.

The most current example, the reverse osmosis system, could be useful against biological terrorism. It could protect us from viruses and lethal bacteria placed by a criminal mind in a small-town water supply network.

---

63 In the case in which the well is too rich in mineral salts.

Microorganisms	Diameter (µm)
Salmonella typhi (typhus)	1.2
Clostridium botulinum (botulism)	1.0
Yersinia pestis (plague)	0.8
Vibrio Cholerae (cholera)	0.5
Poxvirus variolae (smallpox)	0.2
Pores of the Reverse Osmosis membrane	0.0001

From this table it is evident that, for example, the cholera bacillus, whose diameter is 0.5 µm, or the botulinum toxic, which has a diameter of 1.0 µm, would not be able to pass through the pores of the membrane of the reverse osmosis that has a diameter of 0.0001 µm.

To get an idea of the order of magnitude of that measure, consider that the diameter of a red blood cell is equal to 8 µm, whereas that of a hair ranges between 65 and 78 µm.

AN APPROXIMATE KNOWLEDGE OF REALITY

Unfortunately there are some arguments that, for lack of knowledge or due to bias, produce mistrust of the reverse osmosis system. One of the most debated issues is, "Reverse osmosis removes minerals."

To understand the groundlessness of this statement we need to know two essential things:

1. The truth about organic and inorganic minerals;
2. The RDA (Recommended Daily Allowance) of minerals.

THE TRUTH ABOUT ORGANIC AND INORGANIC MINERALS

Recall that there are two types of mineral salts: inorganic and organic. The first minerals are made for plants, the second ones for animals, including humans.

Dr. N.W. Walker says, "Only the living plant has the power to extract inorganic minerals from the soil. The human being cannot derive nourishment from inorganic minerals. If we were shipwrecked on a desert island with no vegetation, we would starve. Although the ground at our feet contains 16 inorganic minerals, our body is unable to absorb them."[64]

Also Paul C. Bragg, a specialist in longevity, says, "The minerals contained in mineral water are inactive. They do not contain enzymes, the essence of life. Nature has provided for breathing life into these minerals through the growth and ripening of plants.

---

64 Walker, N. W., *Water Can Undermine Your Health*. USA, Prescott, AZ: Norwalk Press, 1974.

During the growth of a plant, its roots collect minerals from the soil, then transform them into live organic elements and absorb them into the stem, leaves, seeds, flowers, and fruits."[65]

For example, it would be biologically impossible to nourish the human body by ingesting iron filings or any other form of inorganic iron. The best way to nourish the body with iron is through fresh fruits and raw vegetables. Basically, all the minerals must have a usable form for the body.

Chelation is the process by which minerals adopt their digestible form. Non-chelated minerals cannot be assimilated by our organism. Ninety-nine percent of the minerals contained in water are not chelated; they are inorganic. Only one percent of the minerals in water is organic, which is a very insignificant quantity for our body.

Another thing that is good to remember is that after cooking all organic minerals are transformed into inorganic minerals. This occurs either with water or with food.

THE RDA OF MINERALS

Dr. Henry A. Schroeder, an eminent scholar and a known personality in the world of minerals, said, "The minerals needed by the human body, which are in the water, are insignificant compared to those contained in food. Anyone who merely follows a varied diet, even if it is a diet that is not balanced, absolutely cannot suffer from mineral deficiency."[66]

65 Bragg, P. C., Bragg, P., *Water: The Shocking Truth That Can Save Your Life*. USA, Santa Barbara, CA: Health Science, 2004.
66 Schroeder, H. A., *The Poisons Around Us: Toxic Metals in Food, Air, and Water*. USA, Bloomington, IN: Indiana University Press, 1974.

Even the *American Medical Journal*[67] says, "The minerals that the human body needs are found largely in foods, not in drinking water."

As we just mentioned, the organic minerals found in tap water or bottled water represent only one percent of the total mineral content. For example, a glass of orange juice contains more of these useful minerals than one hundred liters of water.

As a consequence, these minerals can be easily obtained with a proper diet. And, doing so, we would eliminate the risk of ingesting unwanted impurities and inorganic minerals in big quantities.

According to the former chairman of the American Water Quality Association, Mr. Horace Mansfield, in order to get the RDA of some useful minerals for the body an individual should drink:[68]

- 680 glasses of water per day to get the RDA of calcium.
- 1,848 glasses of water per day to get the RDA of iron.
- 168,960 glasses of water per day to get the RDA of phosphorus.

These figures seem to be absurd and unrealistic. Probably the same people who already struggle to drink eight glasses of water a day are those who are worried about getting minerals with water.

It is well known (or at least everyone should know it) that the human body gets the minerals, vitamins, proteins, and everything that is essential, only from the food we eat. In a piece of cheese, a

67 ANON., 1971, "Today's Health," *American Medical Journal*, Volume 49, Issues 7-12.

68 Mansfield, H, "A 'Tasteless' Question: Attention Dealers – Do You Know Distillation?," *WCP*, Vol. 43, Num. 7, July 2001.

sip of milk, or a simple salad leaf, there are more minerals than in hundreds, and sometimes thousands, of liters of water.

To be 100 percent healthy, the human body should be free of inorganic minerals. When pure water enters the human body, it leaves no residue. It is devoid of inorganic salts. It is the perfect drink for internal cleaning and for our health. Pure water is crystal clear thanks to the elimination of all impurities. It is ready and perfect for human consumption, free of all contaminants, including inorganic salts, organic matter, bacteria, and viruses.

The ideal water must have a high capacity to cleanse the body of all the waste products of metabolism. Therefore, it must have a high penetration speed into cells and a high exit speed from them. In other words, it must facilitate rapid water exchange.

A group of Japanese scientists, while studying the causes of the longevity of the population of some centuries-old Japanese islands, discovered that the water consumed by these people was almost devoid of minerals.

WATER NEEDS

The water in the blood transports food and oxygen from the intestines and lungs to the cells. Conversely, waste and carbon monoxide are transported by water (blood and lymph) to kidneys, lungs, and skin, to be expelled, purifying the body. Every day, approximately 6,000 liters of blood circulate through the body. Of this quantity, about 1,600/1,800 liters circulate through the kidneys.

It is easy to see at this point that drinking little water overloads the kidneys, which will make a double effort, and it will take them twice the normal time to filter our little fluid and overloaded blood. But what does it really mean to force the kidneys to work with little water?

It is like driving on a dirty road full of mud. It is obvious that under such conditions, the car would be subject to a bigger effort and it would take much more time driving there than it would take on a paved road. Furthermore, in the same way that a car under these unfavorable conditions would consume more energy, would wear more and would travel fewer miles, so if our kidneys are under hydrated, they will consume more living force, will wear much faster and will work less.

If we drink too little water, the waste to be eliminated will be more and more every day. Thus, it must be removed with less urine, but a more concentrated one. This causes inflammation and sick kidneys.

This biological disaster, however, does not affect only the kidneys, but also all the organs and cells of our body. It will, later on, result in dry skin, wrinkles, weakening of the muscles, liver fatigue, intoxication and acidification of the body, constipation, hemorrhoids, and many other disorders.

By the way, for those who do not know it, drinking too little water causes constipation, which in turn causes hemorrhoids. Do not forget that many diseases or disorders are, in fact, a side effect of other problems.

Many people think that we should drink only when we feel thirsty. Well, that is completely wrong! I must say that, because of the stressful and hectic lifestyles that we have developed with industrialization, many of our instincts have been lost. In fact, many people have lost the stimulus to drink, to stay in the sunlight or to eat healthy.

All these stimuli were (and are) part of our survival instincts. We have not lost them completely. They are simply asleep or atrophied, exactly as it happens to our muscles when we do not use them for a long period of time.

But there is more. The stimulus is in itself a serious alarm. So we do not have to wait and drink until we are thirsty. When we are thirsty, we are probably already very dehydrated.

At the beginning of this chapter I said that under normal conditions the water requirement for an adult is 2.5 liters of water per day. Such water must come from our nutrition in the form of beverages and foods, such as fruits and vegetables. During the day, we should drink at least 1.6 liters of pure water. It is obvious that we should not swallow it all at once, but often and in small quantities, even when we are not thirsty.

FAR FROM HOME

Since tap water is unhealthy, spring water is not accessible to all, and bottled water is too expensive and can be contaminated by both plastic and other contaminants, some may wonder how they can drink water when they are away from home and, therefore, away from a water purifier.

At work, if someone were a manager or an important person, he might install a reverse-osmosis filtration system. In case this is not possible, it is better to take water with us. The biggest problem is not physical but mental. If we pass this psychological obstacle, everything else will be a piece of cake.

In my car, for example, I keep two demijohns of five liters each and, according to my needs, I fill one or both of them with water. There are also larger demijohns with greater capacity. However, the small ones are easier to handle and more comfortable. We can also find demijohns covered in plastic, but I do not recommend them. Wicker demijohns are the best.

Of course, we cannot go to the office with a demijohn of five or ten liters, but if it is necessary, we can easily go to our car and fill a one-liter glass bottle.[69] Please note that I am saying a glass bottle and not a plastic one. Glass, in fact, (better if it is dark) is still the best possible solution for water and food.[70]

The fact remains, however, that it is not very practical to walk around with one or more glass bottles since they are heavy, fragile, and potentially sharp. But I assure readers that, after a while, they will get used to it and this will help toward the improvement and extension of their lives. Water, after food, is the second most important factor in life extension. It is even more important than exercise, which is the third in order. We will discuss this in a forthcoming volume.

Our grandparents did not even consider such kinds of problems. The feeling of discomfort comes from our thought of having to switch from bottles and plastic containers to glass. It is just

---

69 Otherwise you can keep a demijohn also where you work. So you don't have to go away all the time.

70 In fact, the best choice would be using containers and utensils made of wood, as it used to be once upon a time. The wood of these containers and of cutlery must not be colored. They are still used today in many Third World countries.

a psychological problem, nothing more. It is a matter of habit. And I guarantee that your friends will also follow your example after you have told them your point of view.

SOME CLARIFICATIONS

Note that I have not mentioned so far other types of water purifiers. Now, as far as I know, there is no better water purifier in the world than the reverse-osmosis system.[71] For this reason, I considered it unnecessary to take space from more important issues just to illustrate the ineffectiveness of other systems.

I hope that all of us will one day be able to return to drinking tap water again. I would also like that water to be pure and crystal clear, free of contaminants and inorganic salts; in short, a water made on purpose for man and his health.

To make this fact a reality, we all have to get involved personally in not buying or drinking bottled water. We have to participate in some of the campaigns which seek to specify all the possible solutions, such as asking for investments in clean public water for everyone.

Typically, little money is invested in pure tap water. The reason, in part, is that the general opinion thinks that we can drink only bottled water.

Two billion people in the world do not have access to clean water. At the same time, all the cities of the world spend millions of dollars to dispose of plastic bottles that we throw away. Imagine if

---

71 There are some water purification systems that "imitate" reverse osmosis in removing minerals from the water, such as boiling, that I personally do not approve. Even if it is about just the water, boiling may alter its structure. This fact has been demonstrated by the Japanese scientist and researcher Masaru Emoto.

this money was spent on improving the water supply system or, even better, to prevent pollution.

There are many other things we can do to solve this problem. We can put pressure on city governments to restore public drinking fountains and oppose the purchase of bottled water in schools, companies, or throughout the city. This is a huge opportunity for millions of people who can be proactive and can protect not only their wallet, but also the health of their community and the entire planet.

ELISAT ZUBAYRAYEVA

Elisat Zubayrayeva was born February 10, 1882, in the Chechen Republic. The last certain thing about her existence dates back to October 1, 2010, on Grandparents Day, when she was 128 years old.

Elisat holds the title of the oldest person in her country. This fact is unequivocally confirmed by her identity documents.

Granny Elisat spoke about her life in some interviews given to several Russian and Chechen broadcasters. She witnessed a succession of different occasions and remembers almost all the most important events in the history of her country. For example, she remembers what the money looked like at the time of the Tsar—banknotes so large, she says, that there were no more left at the time of Lenin and Stalin

Elisat said that she had nine children, of whom only two sons are still alive.

Until a short time ago, the Chechen grandmother worked in her garden, did domestic chores and was actively involved in family life. Only recently has she begun to be in need of someone to help her. The recent loss of her only daughter was a tragedy that affected her health.

To help her walk, Elisat uses any type of support she can find. But most often she uses a long stick.

Like any woman, Elisat does not like to talk about her age, although she is proud of it. She confessed to reporters that she still sleeps on a hard bed and does not eat products made with flour. She also loves going for long walks outdoors.

She is very optimistic and helpful in the things that she is still able to do. She can sew, spin, braid, and weave. She speaks fluently the Chechnyan and Kyrgyz language.

She often gathers around her grandchildren and great-grandchildren to teach them the Kyrgyz language. Where she lives, in Argun, everyone knows and respects her. There is no party to which Granny is not invited.

Today, in Chechnya, they still follow the ancient tradition of consulting the elders about difficult problems. If someone does not agree with their opinion, it means that person has no respect for the elders.

Considering the same number of inhabitants, Chechnya has more centenarians than Japan; although Chechnya is a poor and undeveloped country compared to the super-developed Japanese society.

Ramzan Digaev, head of the territorial administration of the Federal Statistical Service of the Chechen Republic, in 2008 reported that "In our country there are currently 445 centenarians, among whom 87 exceed 110 years."

If we compare the number of people in the Chechen Republic who are more than 100 years old (445) with the total number of its inhabitants (1,269,100), we can see that there is a centenarian for every 2,852 inhabitants (1,269,100 / 445 = 2,852).

Instead, if we compare the number of people who are more than 100 years old in Japan (30,000) with the total number of its inhabitants, 127,288,419, we find that there is a centenarian for every 4,243 inhabitants. What does this mean?

In Chechnya, there are 35 centenarians for every 100,000 inhabitants (100,000 / 2,852) and in Japan there are only 23 per 100,000 inhabitants. Note that the comparison is made taking into consideration the same number of people. Therefore, in Chechnya, the number of long-living people exceeds by 52 percent that of Japan.

The above example shows that it does not matter in which country of the world we live, or if we live in a rich country or a poor one; if we take all the necessary precautions, we can easily live 120 years because most of the things we do to reach this age we should not be doing anyway, is not an idle pun. By avoiding some things and not adding other things, we can extend our lives by several years: for example, removing table salt, coffee, cigarettes, alcohol, and all industrial non-alcoholic drinks, sugar, refined flour, and refined oils, just to mention a few things.

By now, this idea should be clear: the more processed and

refined foods are the more harmful and toxic to our health they are. In industrialized countries people consume more processed foods, in third world countries people consume more raw products. This is why I say that for longevity, it does not matter where we live. And it is not even important that we are rich or poor. Even though a rich person is, in theory, more likely to live longer than a poor person, this advantage is often lost due to misinformation.

Most of the time, rich people have more trust in doctors, but in doing so they shorten their lives. Many people, unfortunately, have not realized yet that patients are to doctors what buyers are to sellers. In the same way a salesman must do everything possible to get more customers in order to earn his living, so a doctor will do anything for you to be his patient for as long as possible. Even if you are not ill, doctors will still tell you that you are.

By the way, in ancient China doctors were paid as long as the patient remained healthy. But when the patient was ill, the doctors who were treating him would no longer be paid for their service. Today it is exactly the opposite.

During the past few years I followed dozens of cases on TV and in the newspapers that reported how, in a variety of public and private clinics in the world, doctors, in order to get some earnings, used their patients by causing them to believe they had cancer or other diseases. Some underwent unnecessary surgery. How could they do this? They operated on their patients by opening their bodies and then sewing them up. As a consequence, considering that among the patients affected by "cancer" a high rate of survival was recorded, the doctors in question also enjoyed a huge reputation.

One particular case that comes to my mind—just to show what greed and human madness can do—in 2011 a woman had a healthy kidney removed. Unfortunately, this situation can be found in nearly every rich and poor country in the world. Nevertheless, I must say that in poor countries these things happen less frequently. The reasons are obvious: since in these countries people are poor and cannot afford the "treatment," they are also less exposed to the sharks of modern medicine.

But, let's go back to the Granny Elisat.

HER SECRET

In an interview in 2010, Elisat Zubayrayeva said about her old age, "I think that clean air, my healthy lifestyle and physical labor, have contributed to my long life. I never lost my sense of humor and optimism. I have always looked to the future with enthusiasm. And, as you can see, I'm still here."

IS PLASTIC HARMLESS?

We cannot deny the fact that among the innumerable inventions of mankind, plastic has been a major success. In fact, no other material has ever been used on such a large scale. It is omnipresent. It is the factotum of our times. Just look around: plastic, plastic, and more plastic.

Due to its relatively low cost, easy fabrication, and versatility, plastic is used for countless applications, from toys to spacecrafts.

It has changed people's lives. If we peek into our homes, we find plastic everywhere, especially in the kitchen. Here is just a small sample of the multitude of products for which plastic is used: Containers for detergents, packaging, gear, radios and televisions, car and bike parts, electric and thermal insulation of walls, exterior doors, pieces of furniture, windows, gutters, buttons, fuser lamps, transparent covers, objects that mimic ivory, compostable containers, plugs, sockets, domestic appliances, computers, CDs, DVDs, musical instruments, switches, writing materials, laminates, paints, coatings, adhesives, composites, swimming pools, roofing, sport products (canoes, small boats), cosmetics, clothing, shoes, containers for liquids, refrigerator and oven trays, toys, feeding bottles, bottles, food containers, bags, films for food, water pipes, gas pipes, chairs, cutlery, tanks for food use, and many others.

The uses for plastic are almost infinite. So the question arises: is plastic harmless? No, it is not. But this is not the point. It all depends on how and, especially, where it is used.

As long as it does not affect our organism, plastic is welcome. In recent years, this substance has been really overestimated in the sense that it has been accepted without questioning and used even where it should not be used, that is to say, in the kitchen and, unbelievable but true, in hospitals!

In the healthcare environment, not only medicines and solutions are stored in plastic containers, but also I.V. fluids and blood given to patients are kept in plastic bags. Is it healthy to keep blood or drugs in a container made of a mixture of petroleum and highly toxic chemical additives?

According to the pharmaceutical industry and the hospital, yes, it is. On the contrary, for us the answer is no, it is not. The healthiest thing was and still is glass. It is cheap, not toxic, non-polluting and, more importantly, it is 100 percent recyclable.

There is no doubt that plastic is a useful, versatile, durable, and long-lasting material. And in some cases, it lasts even longer than metal. However, it entails disadvantages too. It contaminates the environment and is toxic to our health.

Remember the floating islands of plastic in oceans and seas? They are those huge islands of plastic waste like the one called "Pacific Trash Vortex" that floats on the Pacific Ocean. It continues to grow unabated. So far it is the largest landfill in the world. According to some the island is twice the size of Texas, while for others it might even cover 16 million square kilometers, almost twice the U.S..

In 1997, an American sailor, Charles Moore, discovered the first oceanic landfill near Hawaii. "Every time I came on deck to detect the horizon, I saw a bottle of soap, a bottle cap, or a piece of plastic bobbing. I was in the middle of the ocean and there was not a place where I could move to avoid plastic."

Concerning health, plastic is not good if it comes into contact with food and medicine, but also when we simply breathe its smell, it releases toxins. The Department of Environmental Sciences at the Swedish University of Gothenburg led a study of 83 plastic products in daily use, randomly selected and subject to laboratory analysis, in order to observe the release of potentially dangerous substances in water. The study, which included five of 13 items intended for children, found that one-third of the analyzed products released poisonous substances.. Among them, for example, are toys for the bath and floating toys, together with inflatable arm floats.

"Taking into consideration how much plastic products are spread, how quickly their production has been increased, and the amount of chemicals to which humans and the environment are exposed, it is important to replace the most dangerous substances in plastic products with less dangerous alternatives," pointed out Delilah Lithner, of the Department of Environmental Sciences of the University of Gothenburg.

Researchers have also affirmed that the toxicity of plastic comes mainly from additives and pigments to give special characteristics to the products.

Some substances present in plastics have a chemical structure that, similar to some estrogens, alters the activity of the endocrine system and affects reproductive health. Other substances are not only related to the metabolic syndrome but also affect the reproductive male system, causing serious problems such as cryptorchidism, abnormalities in the penis, and oligospermia.

Apparently, as early as 1936, it was known that the substances found in plastic contaminated the food with which they came in contact. It was also suspected that they modified human sex hormones. A recent study found that these substances are related to prostate cancer.

A small but constant consumption of these substances is particularly dangerous for pregnant women because they distort, in an invisible way but very importantly, the development of the newborn.

These substances cause microscopic changes in the prostate of the fetus, but these are not discernible at birth. The effects appear over the years, in old age, with the appearance of prostate hypertrophy and cancer. Alterations can also cause malformations of the urethra.

The team of Professor Frederick vom Saal, who works at the University of Missouri, has shown that just small amounts of plastic exposure during fetal life are needed.to mess with the male genital system.

Plastic is not as harmless as many people think. The bad thing is that now 80 percent of households in industrialized countries, due to the lack of time or for other reasons, use plastic plates and cups almost daily. An unhealthy trend, I would say, considering all the problems that we face from this behavior.

In fact, plastic plates and glasses produced with derivatives of PVC (polyvinyl chloride) contain highly toxic and carcinogenic substances. People do not realize how many risks they run because of the daily use of these petroleum products. They are unaware that these products contain substances such as phthalates which are highly carcinogenic and particularly are the cause of laryngeal cancer.

Phthalates, contained in plastic plates, tend to leak slowly when they are in contact with hot, alcoholic, or oily foods. This toxic substance is deposited inside the food, and children and adults swallow it.

Phthalates are not the only dangerous component of plastic plates. There it is also the relatively unknown bisphenol A, used in plastics (polycarbonate), in resins, in bottles, tableware (plates, cups, jugs, bowls, and plastic glasses), dishes for microwave ovens, containers, the lining of food cans, and water bottles.

We must also highlight the problem of bioaccumulation, namely, the potential merger of the toxic substances of a plastic plate with an additive or a dye content in the food (for example, a beverage) and with other toxic substances inevitably produced by the contact, for example, of a plastic cup with a hot drink.

Unfortunately, many people are enchanted by what is written on the packaging. They trust blindly in the EU or FDA national security regulations, without knowing that often a politician who puts forward a bill rarely does it in the interest of consumers. Instead, he often seeks to protect the interests of the multinational corporations, disguising or minimizing any health issues that this particular bill would perhaps create over time.

A notable example is the case of aspartame, an artificial sweetener consumed worldwide by more than 200 million people. It is used in more than 6,000 products, including soft drinks, chewing gum, candy, desserts, yogurt, medicines, syrups, and antibiotics for children. Despite having been widely demonstrated at an international level that this substance is carcinogenic, it is still allowed on the market.

In 1981, Donald Rumsfeld, CEO of the pharmaceutical company G. D. Searle, stated in a sales meeting that he would "grease a few screws" to get aspartame approved within the year. Furthermore, he declared that he had used his political influence in Washington, rather than scientific results, to make sure it was approved. And, with the sweetener that was making a large profit, Searle was later bought by Monsanto, notorious for its widespread use of GMOs.

As we can see health always comes in second place with respect to business. Unfortunately, there are many other examples like this one.

People find themselves on the receiving end of all sorts of alleged truths and false certainties for which they will end up paying a high price in terms of their health. Furthermore, they have no possible recourse against those who, with their actions, have been part of the wrongdoing, given the complicity that reigns between politics and multinational companies.

Basically, the problem of plastic dishes for food use is similar to that of aspartame. Both are toxic products. However, they are not withdrawn from the market due to the enormous volume of business that they generate and because all the studies proving their dangerous nature are systematically ignored by the media.

Each person is free to believe and choose whatever he wants. Everyone can choose between being healthy or sick, intelligent or ignorant, winners or losers, predator or prey.

There is a saying, "By force, you can take away something from someone, but you cannot give something by force." I cannot force you to believe what is written in this book. You decide yourself whether to trust my words or the words of a multinational corporation. In my opinion, before you make a choice it is better to consider if there are economic interests at stake.

What about plastic? The first advice is to throw away all the plastic containers in your kitchen used to store food and replace them with glass.

The second advice: Let's behave like our grandmothers. I remember when I was just a child and I went with my grandmother, Sofia, to the grocery store. She carried glass jars for the cheese, cream, fish or any other food she bought. She bought milk and yogurt in glass bottles too. The rule was simple: For wet foods, we used glass containers; for dry foods, cloth or paper bags. Today, as yesterday, almost every supermarket sells food in bulk, in hectograms or kilos.

Third: Whenever possible we should avoid buying food which is stored in plastic. Do not buy fruits or vegetables already packed in plastic. Instead, put them in cloth or paper bags. By doing so, we help nature, the Earth, the environment, and, last but not least, ourselves.

CHAPTER 8

RAW MILK

I had to feed you with milk, not with solid food, because you were
not ready for anything stronger. And you still aren't ready.

The apostle Paul (1 Corinthians 3:2)

The history of milk and dairy products has been intertwined with
the history of humans since they began to domesticate animals. Ten
thousand years ago, the people of Mesopotamia were already trying
to domesticate lactiferous animals. Even then, man was trying to use
and process milk for food purposes.

Archaeological sites dating back to eight thousand years, some
frescoes, and several literary and religious testimonies, have shown
that ancient people consumed milk and cheese. We find indications
of this in ancient Greece, the Roman civilization, in the Bible, in the
writings of Hippocrates, and many others.

In Greek mythology, for example, we see that the discovery of cheese is attributed to the nymphs. It is said that they taught Aristaeus, son of Apollo, the art of milk curdling and transformation.

Even in Roman mythology there are interesting references to milk and cheese. There is the myth of the foundation of the city of Rome by Romulus and Remus, who were nursed by a wolf.

The testimony of Varro Rieti, (116 BC–27 BC) is also very important in the matter. It describes the main types of cheese that were consumed in the first century BC (cow, goat, and sheep, both fresh and seasoned), and they document how in that period the most preferred were those cheeses obtained using rabbit or goat rennet rather than lamb rennet.

PROPERTIES OF RAW MILK

Not many people know that raw milk, and in particular the milk coming from grass-fed animals, has been used not only as food but also as a medicine. There has been talk about its healing effects for at least 2,400 years.

Over the centuries, many doctors of various cultures and traditions have exalted the virtues of milk as valid nourishment and as a medical treatment for numerous ailments. Hippocrates prescribed raw donkey milk for many ills, such as liver problems, edema, epistaxis, poisoning, infectious diseases, plagues, and fevers. The Arab physicians of the Middle Ages prescribed camel milk. And Homer called the Scythians' mighty warriors as *Galactophagi*, i.e., milk eaters.

An American physician, Dr. Porter, did many experiments with milk at the beginning of the last century. In 39 years of clinical practice he obtained excellent results. His patients were suffering from various diseases: heart disease, kidney disease, mental and neurological disorders, ulcers, gastroenteritis, and poisoning (mercury, arsenic, and other heavy metals were also used as medicines at that time).

The American doctor recommended the milk to be fresh, raw, and never subject to boiling and much less to pasteurization, otherwise it would cause the failure of the treatment.

A patient had to take from 1.8 to 3.7 liters of whole milk (at four percent of fat) a day, without consuming other foods, in order not to disturb the digestibility and the curative effect. The treatment lasted for at least a month.

In his writings, Porter claimed that his cure could heal several disorders: fatigue, skin diseases, indigestion, constipation, asthma, hemorrhoids, ulcers, colitis, gout, arthritis, urticaria, cystitis, diarrhea, impotence, sciatica, and hypertension.

Obviously, Dr. Porter's success and other successes of that time were obtained using a type of milk which, apart from not being pasteurized, came from animals kept for most of the year grazing and not locked in concrete stalls, as often happens today. In the indoor-fed cow milk, from cows fed with mash of cereals, certain beneficial qualities are lacking or scarce.

Neither is an integration of dry hay comparable to fresh grass. The milk also has more healing properties if the cows are fed with new spring grass.

In Porter's time, there were also cases of people who lived for years just drinking milk. W. F. Kitzele, from Iowa, was forced to eat only liquid food due to a malformation of the esophagus, and for 42 years he lived a healthy life drinking raw milk only.

COMPARING DIFFERENT TYPES OF MILK

The composition of raw milk varies depending on the animal from which it comes, on its type of food, and on other circumstances. In the table below, we can see some differences between human milk and certain types of milk used by humans:

MILK COMPOSITION ANALYSIS FOR 100 GRAMS

Constituents	Unit of measure	Human	Cow	Goat	Sheep
Water	g	87.5	87.3	88.9	83.0
Proteins	g	1.1	3.2	3.1	5.4
Fats	g	4.2	3.9	3.5	6.0
Carbohydrates	g	7	4.8	4.4	5.1
Energy	kcal	72	66	60	95
Cholesterol	mg	28	11	10	11
Calcium	mg	30	120	100	170

The differences are very small and they are not a problem, as many people believe.[72]

---

72 Some people argue that the milk of various animals is appropriate only to that particular species. This is not true. All the living beings on Earth need more or less the same nutrients: vitamins, enzymes, proteins, carbohydrates, water, and mineral salts. Milk is a biological compound that can be disassembled and reassembled according to the needs of our organism. Therefore, even if in a certain type of milk there is a protein not present in human milk, our body will simply decompose it in amino acids and then will create the protein it needs. Nevertheless, the composition of all types of milk is very similar among them.

WHAT IS RAW MILK?

Many people still do not know exactly what raw milk is. For example, I remember the case of a friend to whom I had explained the benefits of raw milk. Surprisingly, one day she called me from the supermarket to ask me which one was the raw milk.

These were her words, "On the shelf of dairy products, there are at least ten different types of milk, but I have probably found the raw one. It says 'whole milk.' This is it, isn't it?"

"That is not raw milk," I said.

"But on the bottle it says 'fresh,' 'whole' and even 'high quality.'"

So I explained to her that if the bottle is not made of glass and the label does not say raw milk, then it is not raw milk. All the bottles were plastic and on no label was written "raw milk."

What is raw milk then? By definition, raw milk must have been milked on the same day in which it is sold. It must not have undergone any heat treatment or homogenization. But it must have been carefully filtered and brought down to a temperature of 4°C.

The absence of heat treatment, such as pasteurization or sterilization (UHT milk) to which the commonly marketed milk is subject, allows raw milk to integrally preserve its natural characteristics.

Raw milk has always been considered the natural food par excellence, the only one that nature offers to early human life. This food alone is enough to ensure the nutritional requirements in the first and most delicate period of life and growth. Raw milk is, therefore, true milk.

A PERFECT SUBSTANCE

When someone asked a Japanese man of 120 years of age what was the secret of his longevity, he answered, "Every day of my life I drank a glass of raw milk, I ate vegetables, and I rarely ate fatty foods."

But what is so special about raw milk? What is its nutritional and healing power? Is it really a perfect substance?

Yes, indeed, it is. Raw milk is a magical substance. I can say this either from my personal experience or by considering one of the many thousands of people who have been drinking it and still drink it.

It is true that milk is used for children. But it is precisely for this reason that it keeps us young. Because it is used for children, its function is much more important than it seems at first sight.

Considering that since birth onward the existence or not of a species will depend almost entirely on milk, it was created in such a way as to make an organism last as long as possible.

So as long as we continue to drink raw milk, we will not die but live. Regarding milk, it does not matter if the person drinking it is a child or an elderly person; it just keeps us living as long as possible.

THE QUEEN BEE

Worker bees live an average of 50 days, whereas the queen bee lives up to five years. This happens even though the queen bee normally works much more than the working bee. In fact, being the only fertile female in the colony, every day the queen bee lays up to 2,000 eggs. It is a hard job.

Just think about the fact that in order to succeed in her job—

one egg every 43 seconds—the queen bee must not stop, not even for a moment. She also works during the night. She is nourished while working.

And do you know why the queen bee lives on average 36 times longer than the worker bee in spite of working 24 hours a day? Because it is nourished by the bees only with bee "milk," the so-called royal jelly.

Royal jelly is a secretion produced by the hypopharyngeal and maxillary glands of nurse bees. It is used as food for all the bee larvae (only for the first three days of their lives) and for the queen bee for life.

So the queen bee comes from an egg equal to the ones from which all other bee workers come. The only difference is that after three days in the larva stage, the colony decides a particular larva will be the queen bee. She is fed only bees' milk for the rest of her life. Her only nourishment—royal jelly—will be her food for the rest of her life. All other larvae, three days after they are born, will eat the regular food of bees, a mixture of honey and propolis called "beebread."

This also involves, apart from the complete development of the queen bee in relation to the worker bees (sexually immature), an exponential increase in life. In addition, the queen bee is about two times bigger than a worker bee.

In order to lay up to 2,000 eggs per day, the queen bee consumes a quantity of royal jelly which is 80 times her weight.

This phenomenon is also common in other species of insects, for example, in ants, hornets, and wasps. The queens of these colonies live dozens of times longer than their worker insects.

Behold, the belief that hard work shortens our life is again proved to be wrong. If there is some thing that really can influence life span, that thing is nutrition.

With this example, my intention is not to say that people should drink just raw milk all their lives. Neither is it to say that raw milk can extend the life of human beings. However, raw milk can give a person joy, well-being, health, and 30-40 years more of life.

RAW MILK COMPOSITION

Just to simplify the work and to avoid confusion to the reader, unless otherwise specified, all data from now on will refer to cow's milk.

As we already saw in the previous table, the milk of some mammals is very similar to that of human beings with regard to the amount of nutrients. And, as we will see later, its quality is very similar as well.

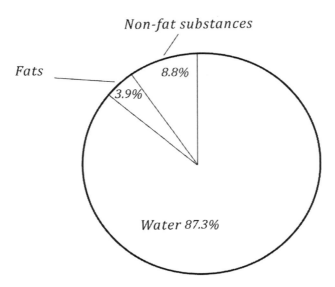

CREATED TO NOURISH

Milk is one of the few foods in nature whose sole function is nourishment. There are six classes of nutrients present in milk— carbohydrates, proteins, fats, water, vitamins, and minerals—that are perfectly proportioned to the nutrients that constitute our body.

Apart from milk, there are other natural foods whose sole function is nourishment. They are honey, royal jelly, and, in part, the egg. The latter is composed mainly of nutrients necessary for the development and growth of the embryo during the period of incubation. For hens, it is 21 days. This is why I consider milk, eggs, and honey essential foods for humans.

Now let us look more closely at the elements present in raw milk and see what makes this food so complete. As mentioned earlier, it is made up mainly of water, then of non-fat substances such as carbohydrates, proteins, minerals, vitamins, and, finally, fats.

WATER

In raw milk, water is the most abundant nutrient. We have already discussed its importance in the chapter "The Secrets of Water."

Since raw milk must not be filtered as we do with the water, it is essential that cows drink only clean, uncontaminated water. Of course, the water contained in milk is filtered in the best possible way by the organs of the cow. But this happens only as long as the cow is young and healthy. In the long run, when the cow is full of waste and toxins, her milk will be inexorably contaminated. I am not saying that cows must necessarily drink filtered water. What I mean is simply that it would be enough, and also the best thing, to give the cows water to drink from artesian wells.

Some people might wonder why milk is so rich in water. The answer is, to maintain the proper water balance of infants or of those who drink it. About 70 percent of the human organism is made up of water that must be continually replenished?

BUTTERFAT

Butterfat is the most complex fat in nature. In it, more than 400 different fatty acids have been identified. Nevertheless, only 14 of them have a concentration that is above one percent and they alone constitute more than 90 percent of the total fat. Butterfat is made up about 65 percent of saturated acids, 30 percent of monounsaturated acids and five percent of polyunsaturated fatty acids.

Fatty acid composition of cow's milk			
Saturated acids	**(%)**	**Unsaturated acids**	**(%)**
Palmitic acid	27	Oleic acid	24
Myristic acid	11	Linoleic acid	2.7
Stearic acid	10	Palmitoleic acid	2.5
Burytic acid	4	Linolenic acid	1.8
Lauric acid	4	**Subtotal**	**31**
Capric acid	3	**Other acids**	**6.2**
Caproic acid	2.5		
Caprylic acid	1.3		
Subtotal	**62.8**	**Total**	**100**

The table shows the average data recorded on samples of cow's milk from 60 Italian farms. For practical reasons, I have included only the data of the top 12 most prevalent fatty acids in milk fat.

From this datum we can see that eight saturated acids form about 62.8 percent of the fatty acids. Four unsaturated acids represent 31 percent of them. Finally, all other acids, i.e., the remaining 388 acids, saturated and unsaturated, make up 6.2 percent of the total.

Saturated acids are those present in greater quantities. Is this good or bad? It depends. If the milk has not undergone any heat treatment or skimming, it is a good thing. But that is not the point. The most important thing is that the fatty acids in milk have a very complex and precise structure. They are not an accumulation of chaotic fat. Every acid, in fact, has a specific function. Apart from transporting through our organism several vitamin factors, the acids are used by the body for the production of hormones and for the construction of tissues, such as nervous tissues.

Another milk quality is represented by its variability. Just as the sun's electromagnetic waves change from morning to night and from season to season, also the fatty acid composition of milk does not remain constant during the entire lactation period.

For this reason, an infant formula can never have the characteristics of true milk. Raw milk is dynamic and alive, whereas the artificial one is dull and dead. Never give your child infant formula. Actually, the latter should not even be called milk.

Each fatty acid in milk plays a number of key roles within our body. Their roles range from the formation of cell walls and hormones for the transport of soluble vitamins to the storage of energy and the transfer of the unique and delicious flavor of milk and butter.

Blaming fat for causing heart disease is like blaming water because it does not flow when the pipes are blocked. The fats in the arteries are the effect, not the cause. The cause may be something other, for example, refined foods, salt, hydrogenated and processed fats, sugar, or cooked food. If a landslide blocks the passage of cars on the highway, we cannot blame the cars because they are deposited on the artery of the highway for 20 km.

We must consider that prior to the hydrogenation process to make solid oils, very few people were dying from heart disease. In any case, we will discuss oils and fats in detail in the next volume.

Milk also contains two essential fatty acids, i.e., those that the body cannot synthesize and which must be introduced through the diet to keep the body in good health. We are talking about the alpha-linolenic acid, an Omega-3, and linoleic acid, belonging to the group of the Omega-6.

Conjugated linoleic acid (CLA) is an Omega-6 acid, a polyunsaturated and heavy fat that seems to be a promising factor against many diseases. It is found in abundance in the milk of pasture-fed cows.

I have to specify something about trans-fatty acids. They are of two types: trans-fatty acids produced artificially and those that are found naturally in animal fats. Even if they have the same name, they are not equal. As a matter of fact, there is a huge difference between the effects on health caused by trans-fatty acids obtained from the industrial processing of vegetable oils and the effects produced by trans-fatty acids naturally present in animal fats such as milk or eggs. The latter have a fatty acid profile very different from the former.

While the natural ones have positive effects on health, the artificial ones are harmful. They cause heart disease and cancer, while natural trans-fatty acids do the opposite; they inhibit cancer and protect us from cardiovascular disease.

The CLA also strengthens the immune system, increases our metabolic rate, helps remove body fat, promotes the action of the muscles, reduces the impact of food-allergic reactions, and reduces insulin resistance.

Raw milk derived from pasture-fed cattle contains a quantity of linoleic acid from three- to-five times higher than milk derived from cows not raised primarily on a forage diet.

Another fatty acid that is found in milk is the palmitoleic acid. Recent studies coordinated by the Italian geneticist Annibale Puca have shown that in the children of long-living people there is a very high level of palmitoleic acid at the cell membrane level. The sensitivity of the insulin receptors of the liver and muscles seems to depend on this acid.

MILK PROTEINS

Proteins are complex molecules formed by long chains of amino acids bound together by peptide bonds. We can compare amino acids to building blocks for protein construction, and peptide bonds to the glue that holds them together.

Proteins contribute to the formation of 20 types of different amino acids. Our organism synthesizes just 12 of them. The remaining eight must be introduced through food and are therefore defined essential amino acids. Depending on the type, the number, and order of sequence in which the different amino acids are bound, it is possible to obtain an infinite number of proteins.

Cow's milk contains all 20 amino acids that humans need. About 80 percent of the proteins are caseins, and the remaining 20 percent are whey proteins. The latter are found in the serum, the liquid part of milk, which is separated from the curd during cheese production.

The caseins, from the Latin *caseus*, "cheese," are a family of phosphoproteins (αS1, αS2, β, κ). These proteins are commonly found in mammals' milk. They constitute 80 percent of the proteins in cow's milk and between 20 percent and 45 percent in human milk.

Casein is an important component of cheese and, as a food, provides amino acids, carbohydrates, enzymes, calcium, and phosphorus.

The FSANZ, Food Standards Australia New Zealand, maintains, "The protein β (A2) of casein provides protection against autistic disorders and diseases such as schizophrenia, diabetes, and heart disease." According to a study of the Australian Dairy Council, casein has anti-mutagenic effects.

The biological value of caseins is lower than that of whey proteins, which instead are richer in essential amino acids. Furthermore, whey proteins play several important physiological roles for our health.

Key enzymes (specialized proteins), inhibitors of enzymes, immunoglobulins (antibodies), proteins bound to metals, proteins bound to vitamins, and many growth factors are part of the whey proteins. They are easy to digest but very heat sensitive.

Some cow milk proteins			
Casein protein	(%)	**Whey protein**	(%)
α (s1)-casein	30.6	α-lactalbumin	3.7
α (s2)-casein	8.0	β-lactoglobulin	9.8
β-casein	28.4	Serum albumin (BSA)	1.2
κ-casein	10.1	Immunoglobulins	2.1
		Proteose-peptone	2.4
Subtotal	**77.1**	**Subtotal**	**19.2**

Proteins are among the more complex organic compounds and are the fundamental constituents of all animal and plant cells. In an adult man, the body proteins amount to about 12 kg.

In the serum, as I mentioned earlier, are the main milk proteins, the elite, so to speak. In addition to the above-cited proteins, in the serum we also find the famous lactoferrin growth factors, and many other minor enzymes and proteins. Let us examine some of them.

IMMUNE FACTORS

The term "immune factors" identifies all those substances that help our bodies defend themselves against the aggression of various external agents such as viruses, bacteria, fungi, protozoa, etc. Some immune factors have well-defined functions. For example, they stimulate the activation of a particular defense mechanism while others operate on a more generic level, giving defensive effectiveness to our entire immune system or to a part of it.

Some of the most important immune factors in bovine milk include immunoglobulins, proline-rich polypeptides, lactoferrin, cytokines, some enzymes, glycoproteins, and inhibitors of trypsin, lysozyme, lymphocytes, oligo and polysaccharides, and glycoconjugates.

We will analyze only two immune factors in order not to get weighed down with detail because we do not need a medical degree to drink a glass of raw milk.

IMMUNOGLOBULINS (IG):

Immunoglobulins are a very complex class of milk proteins. They are the main immune factors present in bovine milk. They are commonly called antibodies, as the body normally produces them for defensive purposes when foreign substances (antigens) are present within it.

In general, the functions attributed to immunoglobulins include the neutralization of toxins, viruses, and bacteria in the bloodstream and the lymphatic system. Immunoglobulins are large protein molecules made up of chains of hundreds of amino acids and can work together or separately to destroy antigens. Some of them circulate in the blood, others in the lymphatic system; others reside in the mucous membranes and act as a barrier against the invasion of harmful foreign agents. Immunoglobulins are present in all mammals, including man. They can be divided into several classes: IgA, IgD, IgE, IgG and IgM, each of which has different specific functions.

Immunoglobulins play an important role in the body's defenses against external attacks. In recent years, their role is becoming increasingly crucial due to the onset of resistance phenomena to antibiotics in the bacteria.

LACTOFERRIN:

Lactoferrin is an iron-binding protein that is found in high concentrations in milk. There are more than two thousand published studies on its biological functions. These studies clearly show that this protein, apart from transporting iron, is a natural antioxidant and a powerful activator of natural-killer cells. It plays an important role in the defense against tumors. It regulates granulopoiesis, cellular cytotoxicity, cytokine production, and the growth of certain cells in vitro. Furthermore, it has an immune action and inhibits the release of histamine from mast cells.

Lactoferrin has important anti-viral, anti-inflammatory, and anti-bacterial properties. It can protect the body from candidiasis, chronic fatigue syndrome, herpes, and other infections. The dynamic action of lactoferrin is unique because it is able to destroy bacteria and to supply iron to our bodies. What lactoferrin does in practice is to free the bacteria of iron, preventing them from reproducing, and making iron available for the functions of our organism—first of all, the function of supplying oxygen to all our cells.

Studies carried out in France show that in persons to whom bovine lactoferrin was administered there was an increase of immunoglobulins IgA and IgG when compared to the control group.

There are also some studies that show that bovine lactoferrin inhibits carcinogenesis in the colon, bladder, tongue, esophagus, and the lungs. Other studies report that lactoferrin may be used for the treatment of the hepatitis C virus and as a preventive agent of liver cancer.

Lactoferrin is also produced by the exocrine glands of the digestive, respiratory, and reproductive systems. However, with increasing age, stress, and other negative factors, its production by the body tends to decrease.

Bovine lactoferrin is made up of 689 amino acids, whereas the human lactoferrin is made up of 691 of them. The sequence identity is 69 percent. Note that the first 52 amino acids forming bovine lactoferrin are, from the functional point of view, identical to those present in human lactoferrin. The rest of the molecule is similar.

Edward N. Baker of the University of Auckland, New Zealand, during the sixth International Conference on Lactoferrin in 2003, stated, "Although the antiviral and antibacterial activity of lactoferrin and its ability to modulate immune responses are reliable, we are still far from understanding its mechanisms at a molecular level."

Another characteristic of lactoferrin in bovine milk is its ability to inhibit the accumulation of oxidized LDL cholesterol at the artery wall level and thus the formation of those plaques that are mainly responsible for the onset of arteriosclerosis.

In this regard, a study reports that bovine lactoferrin would be even more effective than the human one in inhibiting the formation of the bond between the modified LDL cholesterol and macrophages, interacting directly with this type of cholesterol. In this way, the deposit and accumulation of macrophages containing oxidized LDL cholesterol on the walls of arteries would actually be prevented.

Recapitulating, the immune factors present in bovine milk provide an incredible protective efficacy thanks to their surprising concentration which is twenty times greater than that of human milk.

UPDATE YOUR ANTIVIRUS

The antivirus is a type of software which is able to detect and remove computer viruses or other malicious programs from your computer. It is equipped with a database containing the "identikit," namely, the typical patterns of each virus (trojans, worms, malware, etc.).

The scheme of the virus, also called *virus signature*, is made up of a specific number of instructions. To protect your computer from one of these malicious softwares, the antivirus must check whether one of these sequences is present in the files or the memory. The success of this research technique is based on the constant updating of virus signatures within its database.

From the immunological point of view, the consumption of raw milk can be compared to the updating of the computer antivirus. In fact, milk is rich in natural substances that work by "teaching" the immune system to identify pathogens that attack our bodies every day.

We must remember that, just as the computer antivirus is able to remove only the viruses it can recognize—and thus all the new viruses can pass completely unnoticed and act without the intervention of the antivirus—so our immune system can identify and destroy first of all only the harmful bacteria, fungi, parasites, toxins, or viruses that it recognizes.

A key feature of the immune system is, therefore, the ability to distinguish between endogenous or exogenous structures that are not dangerous and therefore may or must be preserved, and the endogenous or exogenous structures that instead are proved to be harmful to the organism and therefore must be eliminated.

The immune system has to fulfill three basic functions in order to keep the body in good health whenever it comes into contact with a pathogen. First, it must recognize the pathogen as a threat to the organism. Second, it must attack and destroy the threat. And finally, it has to remember that specific pathogen so that it can quickly get rid of the pathogen in case it comes back.

It is true that many immunological memory molecules have been transmitted to us from breast milk, but it must be said that conditions have changed since then. In fact, many bacteria and viruses are constantly changing.

The immune factors that we received from our mothers when we were children helped form and strengthen our immune system and adapt it to the challenges of that time. Today, more than ever, we are exposed to new immunological challenges, while our immune system is weakened. For this reason, strengthening our immune system can be decisive for a long life and good health.

For individuals suffering from specific diseases, the administration of the correct molecule of raw milk may provide the missing link that will allow the immune system to frame and destroy the pathogen and mitigate the symptoms of the disease.

We should not forget that many small children have received little breast milk, or did not receive it at all.

GROWTH FACTORS

Growth factors are compounds whose main effects are the promotion of health through the construction, maintenance, and repair of bones, muscles, nerves, and cartilage. They actively participate in the stimulation of fat metabolism, in the regulation of protein metabolism during fasting, in the maintenance of proper blood sugar levels, in the regulation of the substances in the brain that control our mood, and in the healing of tissues. A further advantage related to the presence of growth factors seems to be their anti-ageing action, particularly in the case of the skin.

Some of the growth factors contained in bovine milk are the epidermal growth factor (EGF), fibroblast growth factor (FGF), transforming growth factors (TGF A & B), and insulin-like growth factors I and II (IGF-I and IGF II).

There is no need to analyze all the growth factors, so we will take into consideration only the last one mentioned, namely, the insulin-like growth factor I and II (IGF-I and IGF II). If a reader is interested in knowing in depth the function of each milk element, he may check the vast bibliography on milk. Even on the Internet we can find websites dealing with this topic.

The only risk with regard to either the books or the Internet is to come across information aimed at defaming raw milk, or milk in general. What should you do in these cases? Should you open the book and see what types of milk the author talks about? Of course not. We are not interested in a text that speaks badly of pasteurized milk and dairy products (cheese, yogurt, butter) because we already know that this is bad. Neither are we interested in texts that slander milk in general. We can easily recognize these kinds of books by their titles, for example, *Milk Is Bad*, or *Milk, a Food to Avoid*.

INSULIN-LIKE GROWTH FACTORS I AND II:
These types of proteins influence the utilization of fats, proteins, and sugars by the body. They stimulate the immune system and promote repair mechanisms and cell growth.

Since all cells of the body are equipped with a receptor for the IGF-II, this growth factor can help each cell heal or reproduce. In particular, the IGF-I is one of the few known substances capable of stimulating the growth of and repairing DNA and RNA.

Its restorative properties make the IGF-I one of the most powerful anti-ageing substances. The IGF-I is a substance capable of arousing considerable interest among bodybuilders because it is able to stimulate the growth of muscles without favoring the storage of fat.

According to the results of some studies, it seems that IGF-I lowers the levels of LDL cholesterol and increases those of HDL cholesterol. A survey dated 1990 showed that IGF-I exerts an alternative effect to that of insulin on glucose transport in the muscles. It could be a potential treatment against high blood sugar and possibly a partial substitute for insulin—probably useful in the reduction of the doses indicated for patients suffering from insulin-dependent diabetes. The IGF-I has also some benefits on the immune system since it stimulates the production of T cells

The main reason for the presence of growth factors IGF-I and II in milk is the promotion of the rapid development of the tissues through the stimulation of protein synthesis in human newborns.

In adults, the IGF-I and II factors play a role of great importance since they are involved in cell proliferation and in the regulation of repair, of growth, and of differentiation of tissue. In athletes who undergo particularly intense and frequent training, it is obvious that tissue repair is even more relevant.

The growth factor IGF-I is released from many tissues in the body and may exert its effect on most of our cells. The main organs that synthesize IGF-I are the heart, lungs, kidneys, liver, spleen, pancreas, small and large intestines, testes, ovaries, brain, bones, the pituitary gland, and the placenta.

The majority of IGF-I is secreted by the liver in response to the signal launched by the human growth hormone (hGH). The principal tissues that receive it are the muscles, cartilage, bones, liver, kidneys, nerves, skin, and lungs.

The growth factor IGF-I assists the cells during cell division, DNA synthesis, and differentiation. In general, we can say that the IGF-I reports an anabolic signal to cells regulating their division and specialization.

In particular, in muscle this anabolic signal is concentrated in moments of stress or when some damage has occurred. In general, we can say that IGF-I promotes not only the synthesis of muscle tissue, but also of bone. IGF-I also acts as part of the nervous system and plays a role of considerable importance in the growth and development of nerve cells.

Furthermore, IGF-I keeps an efficient communication at neuromuscular joints' level, which is the primary location in which the real cooperation between the nerve and muscle cells occurs. It is also believed that the factor IGF-I is able to return to the older or fatigued cells an adequate level of activity, thereby allowing the tissue to maintain its usual performance.

The administration of raw cow's milk during training sessions aimed at enhancing the speed and strength of athletes can increase the natural concentration of IGF-I in their blood.

It is interesting to know that the normal levels of IGF-I in our bodies tend naturally to decrease with ageing, stress, frequent contact with toxins in the environment, and the gradual acquisition of a more and more sedentary lifestyle. Therefore, the regular intake of cow's milk can help integrate the growth factors necessary for our body. Furthermore, it is connected to a balanced appetite and a significant decrease of body fat.

MILK ENZYMES

Enzymes are biological catalysts that can accelerate a chemical reaction. All enzymes are proteins, but not all proteins are enzymes.

Raw milk contains about 60 known enzymes, each of which is essential for several fundamental reactions. Some of them are naturally present in milk and others come from beneficial bacteria–lactobacillus that grow in milk. This aspect is one of the most important with regard to the food properties of milk and the consequent reduction in the occurrence of diseases.

The enzymes present in food help our organism with digestion. When we eat something that contains enzymes useful for digestion, our pancreas has to work a lot less. The amylase, lactase, lipase, and phosphatase present in raw milk react with the starch, with the lactose, with fats (triglycerides), and with phosphorus, making the milk more digestible and releasing key minerals. Other enzymes, such as catalysis, lysozyme, and lactoperoxidase, help protect milk from unwanted bacterial infection, making it safer to drink.

MILK CARBOHYDRATES

Lactose is the first carbohydrate that the majority of mammals consume from infancy. It is made up of two simple sugars, glucose and galactose, which both form a disaccharide.

Cow's milk contains approximately five percent lactose, which represents 98 percent of all the sugars present in milk. Thanks to its reasonably low glycemic index, lactose is better tolerated by people with diabetes.

Some people, however, have difficulty digesting lactose. This disorder is generated by the production shortfall from the intestinal cells of the duodenum of the enzyme lactase, assigned to the breaking down of the lactose into glucose and galactose which, in this form, can then be absorbed.

The poor digestion of lactose, defined as lactose intolerance, is characterized by excessive production of gas within the intestinal lumen, from abdominal cramps to diarrhea. Some think that it is a disease, but the good news is that actually it is not. More precisely, it is a temporary disturbance which can be corrected.

What happens to a muscle if we do not use it for months or years? It atrophies. When our body sees that a muscle or an enzyme is no longer needed, it puts the muscle in stand-by mode and disables or decreases the production of the enzyme.

Nevertheless, the muscle is not permanently deleted because tomorrow it is likely to be needed. In the case of the enzyme, the matter is even simpler: to activate or cease its production, our body simply has to activate certain genes and deactivate others.

Why then do we become lactose intolerant? The answer is

obvious. The production of the lactase enzyme necessary to digest the lactose decreases gradually with the decrease in the consumption of raw milk or in the absence of constant consumption.

As we get older, lactase levels often decrease significantly. This is not a problem if we consume raw milk because it already contains this enzyme. But when we consume heat-treated milk products, since the enzyme of the food is no longer active and because the sufficient quantity of lactase to break down lactose is lacking, unpleasant symptoms such as swelling and diarrhea appear. However, raw milk, thanks to the live lactobacilli, has the lactase produced by the bacteria still intact so that people can easily tolerate it.

The bacteria naturally present in milk—lactobacilli or lactic ferments—in addition to enriching raw milk with enzymes, vitamins, and mineral salts, transform the lactose into lactic acid, which in turn has inhibitory effects on many harmful species of bacteria. In addition, the lactic acid increases the absorption of calcium, phosphorus, and iron, and makes milk proteins more digestible.

Another way to enjoy the benefits of milk products while eliminating the drawbacks of lactose digestion consists of eating fermented products such as yogurt and kefir. During the fermentation process, the useful microbes described above "digest" almost all the lactose, turning it into lactic acid, which is a powerful antimicrobial agent.

Cheeses made from raw milk are more flavorful and, for the reasons mentioned above, do not contain lactose. Most of the lactose is consumed during the fermentation process.

Some people think they are allergic to milk. This is true only in part. The possible milk allergies are triggered by certain proteins

250

that have undergone a heat treatment by pasteurization or boiling, so those who consume raw milk cannot have allergies to milk.

VITAMINS

Raw milk is also an excellent source of fat-soluble and water-soluble vitamins. In order to take all of them, we must make sure to drink only raw whole milk because vitamins are lost in the process of skimming and/or pasteurization.

Basically, there is no need to add anything to raw milk to make it whole or better, especially in milk from grass-fed cows. No vitamins and no minerals need to be added. It is already a complete food.

The heating of raw milk destroys many of its nutrients, in particular enzymes and the important fat-soluble vitamins A and D. The minerals and synthetic vitamins added after pasteurization by the food industry do nothing but tarnish even more the already denatured milk.

Two of the most important vitamins in milk, riboflavin (vitamin B_2) and vitamin A, play a number of important functions in our organism.

The first vitamin, which was originally named lactoflavin because of its presence in considerable quantities in milk, is a constituent of several enzyme systems involved in cellular redox processes and is involved as well in many other reactions, including the synthesis of folic acid.

Vitamin A is indispensable for vision and for cell differentiation and is therefore necessary for growth, reproduction, and the integrity of the immune system.

MINERAL SALTS

Here we come to the last class of nutrients, mineral salts. Unlike those of water, the minerals in raw milk are organic, i.e., organically bound to the enzymes.

In the chapter "The Secrets of Water," we talked about the importance of minerals being organic and not inorganic, because from the latter man cannot be nourished.

Raw milk contains a wide selection of mineral salts, ranging from calcium and phosphorus to particular microelements, the function of which has not been fully clarified yet.

Needless to say, with pasteurization all minerals contained in milk become inorganic minerals. Milk, like any other genuine food, can be a source of health when consumed raw, and a source of disease if consumed pasteurized or boiled. It is better to completely avoid milk rather than drink pasteurized milk. That's because pasteurized milk not only does not help our body, but even pollutes it and makes it sick.

Even though our body can tolerate certain cooked foods, the same thing does not apply to milk. In fact, milk is a food that is too complex to play with fire. Some toxic mushrooms,[73] after boiling become edible, whereas raw milk, after cooking or pasteurization, becomes toxic.

---

73 This example demonstrates that in these fungi it is not a chemical substance which is toxic, but a biological one, i.e., a substance that is alive. Most of the time it is an enzyme inhibitor or an enzyme. While the chemicals do not change after boiling, the biological ones do. In our case, boiling destroys the enzyme of the fungus that is harmful to us, making it inactive. Other things happen with all the other enzymes when they are heat treated.

PASTEURIZATION KILLS MILK

Undoubtedly, today commercial milk, namely the pasteurized and homogenized kind, is for many people a source of health problems such as colds, inflammation, water retention, dermatitis, allergies, diarrhea, constipation, and so on.

Yet, once milk was used to treat many of these same disorders. What happened? It is not difficult to imagine that the main cause of the loss of the health benefit virtues of milk is due primarily to pasteurization. Other causes are related to the way in which animals are raised and fed.

We learned in school that pasteurization was introduced by the French scientist Louis Pasteur and that it consists of heating foods at temperatures that exceed 80°C in order to destroy the bacteria. It seems to be a good thing per se. Instead, with pasteurization, foods lose much of their nutritional value and affect our health. This fact has been demonstrated by numerous researches and experiments.

One of these experiments was published in the Oxford journal *Mind and Matter*.[74] "In an agricultural school in Scotland, some experiments were carried out to monitor the effects of nursing calves with pasteurized milk and raw milk respectively. From the very first day of their life, eight calves were fed with pasteurized milk, and eight others with raw milk. Two animals in the first group died after the first month, while with another of the calves it was decided to stop the experiment in order not to kill him. The fourth calf died two days after the end of the experimental period, while the rest were saved with the administration of raw milk. The calves of the second group,

---

74 "Mind and Matter," n. 6/1958.

which did not receive degraded milk, were all in good health."

Two American scholars, Potenger and Simonsen, tested nutrition with pasteurized milk on cats, articulating studies involving more than three generations of cats.[75] The cats that were fed with raw milk grew normally, while those fed with pasteurized milk developed a severe form of rickets which later killed them. All the cats which did not receive raw milk from the first generation had abortions.

The animals showed abnormalities in behavior, becoming aggressive, scratching and biting. In 53 percent of the animals, the thyroid gland was undeveloped, while the third generation of animals were almost all deformed.

As the above studies indicate, milk loses its benefits and its nutritional qualities immediately after it is heated or boiled. The famous Canadian biologist H. Tobe wrote in his book *Enzymes, the Spark of Life*,[76] that through heating and pasteurization during food processing, all the enzymes of vital importance to us are destroyed. As a result, the main elements of milk, in particular calcium, iron, and phosphorus, can no longer be assimilated and metabolized by the body except in small quantities. All that is left forms an accumulation of waste in our body. The disease germs, swarming everywhere, find a fertile ground for development in the blood full of the waste of pasteurized products. This is how a disease originates.

In the words of the British researcher J. H. Oliver, written in his book *Proven Remedies*,[77] "Why is a dry twig attacked by germs and

75 "Kneipp Journal," n. 2/1972.
76 Tobe, J. H., Enzymes, the Spark of Life, Canada, Ontario: Modern Publications, 1966.
77 Oliver, J. H., Proven Remedies, United Kingdom, London: Thorson, 1949.

bacteria, and not a healthy one, which is full of juice and life? Because the bacteria have been created precisely to remove the accumulated residues, and thus they play an important role in nature. Yet, as soon as they find a deposit of waste in the blood and attack cell tissue, we blame them for the suffering they caused even though they are not the ones that caused the disease."

To be sure of that fact and to prove it, Professor Rudolf Emmerich[78] swallowed an entire vial of cholera which, of course, did not cause him any damage.

A very careful mom, in the nutrition of her child, decided that her baby would drink raw milk only from a certain cow, owned by a friend of hers. She was sure she could trust the honesty of her friend.

After a while, it was discovered that the cow was suffering from tuberculosis and that the disease was at an advanced stage. Perhaps the child had swallowed millions of germs of tuberculosis. Were they harmful to him? Not at all! Drinking raw milk and eating other raw vegetables, the child had developed a very strong constitution so that the bacteria had not found a favorable and benevolent environment for their development.

Z. H. Oven added that "raw milk is a masterpiece diet." If pasteurized, it becomes "a door wide open to disease and death."

All these tests show that both boiling and pasteurization of milk are completely useless. They not only affect our health, but millions of dollars are wasted to devalue food.

---

78 Science, vol. 5. Jan, New York, 1885.

RAW MILK VENDING MACHINES

In some countries, the law forbids the sale of raw milk. Neither are peasants allowed to sell it. The ignorance of many people has allowed some profiteers to vote on a similar bill.

Luckily, in some countries such as Italy, Germany, France, and others, the law still allows the sale of raw milk in vending machines after it has been cooled down to 4°C. The vending machines are managed by computers that keep the temperature under control.

The milk is fresh, milked a couple of hours before—good, creamy, filtered, and controlled in accordance with the latest food and health techniques. It is tasty and comes strictly from cows reared according to the ancient tradition. All a person needs to do is insert coins into the machine and fill a bottle; after that he can drink it immediately or take it home and keep it in the refrigerator for 3–4 days.

The direct sale of raw milk has a double economic advantage as it is beneficial to both producers and consumers.

The consumer spends on average 30 percent less than in the supermarket and the producer gets a profit of at least twice as much as when he sells the milk to the industry.

Therefore, raw milk sold directly to consumers is an important source of income for the farmer. In fact, for a liter of milk sold to the milk industry, he receives a price that ranges from €0.32 to 0.42; while from the vending machines one liter of raw milk is sold on average for €1. This means that a farmer could earn more than double from the vending-machine milk. Besides, the consumer has much to gain too, since in supermarkets pasteurized milk costs from €1.50 to €1.80 per liter.

The price of milk paid to the producer is the same as it was 15 years ago. That is why we sometimes hear on TV that farmers throw milk away. All this is certainly the result of a short-sighted policy toward milk producers.

Thanks to direct sales and a fair price for the milk, producers will have every incentive to keep their milk as healthy as possible and their animals in very good condition.

The advantages of the raw milk vending machines, in addition to the intrinsic characteristics of raw milk rather than pasteurized milk, are:

1. The milk is always fresh daily. In fact, this type of milk is milked every day between 5 a.m. and 6 a.m. and, after being filtered and cooled down to 4°C, it is transported to the vending machines between 8 and 10 a.m. The next day, when the farmer brings the fresh milk of that day, the milk remaining from the previous day will be withdrawn. For this reason, the raw milk that we find in the vending machines could have been milked from a minimum of two to three hours to a maximum of 24 hours. The pasteurized "fresh" milk in the supermarket, even if it was just brought to the shelves, will have been around at least two to three days, whereas the long-conservation milk may easily have been around for two to three months.

2. It does not contaminate either the purchaser or the environment. Plastic containers hurt both the milk and the milk drinker. A simple glass bottle can be used for a lifetime. Just think how many plastic bottles or Tetrapak containers are

thrown away! In 2008, in Italy, where there are about 1,000 vending machines, there has been an annual environmental savings of at least 30 million unused bottles, namely, a total of about 3,000,000 kg of packaging.

3. It is a zero km milk. The distance between the place where the milk is produced to the vending machine is normally only a few kilometers. Consequently, in this way, we have an environmental savings by eliminating transportation to the processing industry, the next transportation for marketing, and that of the recall for unsold products. In some cases pasteurized milk is transported thousands of miles away. For example, the milk from Germany ends up in Italy, or the milk from Siberia is brought to Moldova.

4. It draws the producer nearer to the consumer.

5. Fresh milk is better controlled than pasteurized milk.

6. It is available 24 hours a day.

7. There are many other advantages to having vending-machine milk.

A CHILD'S GAME

A person can equip himself with a glass bottle, take a coin, place it into the slot of the self-service vending machine, and finally take home the milk. The law says the milk should be consumed within three days. However, those people who do not have the time to go and get the milk very often, as it happens to me, can keep it in the refrigerator at 4°C safely for a week. In fact, several years ago, before the vending machines were invented, I had to go to a farm outside the city to get raw milk. Since I did not have time to go every day, I'd buy enough milk for the whole week.

Now things have changed. We can find automatic machines either in malls or outdoors in the streets, and they are always open 24 hours a day. Every self-respecting country should have a website with a map showing where all the vending machines of raw milk are located. For example, in Italy the website is, http://www.milkmaps.com.

As a curiosity, raw milk never goes bad, even if kept out of the refrigerator for a month. What happens is that after about a week it separates into two distinct parts, the cream above and the curds below, which is a kind of yogurt. Pasteurized milk can cause poisoning if consumed after the deadline. While raw milk is alive and has an immune enzyme structure, the pasteurized milk is dead along with its defenses.

To make a comparison, when an animal is alive it can defend itself from the bacteria, except in special cases. But once it is dead it is devoured in a week by bacteria and worms.

THE RISKS OF RAW MILK

Not bad, someone would object, if there are no risks. What are the risks? From the examples presented previously, we see that the risks are greater and more numerous in the case of pasteurized milk. In the Caucasus, Bulgaria, and other Eastern states, raw milk and curdled milk are the basic foods and no one thinks that they entail any risk. If so many people in these countries live more than a hundred years, they can only thank raw milk!

The fear of being ill is so great that it wins despite all the benefits of raw milk. Those people who tell us to beware of unpasteurized milk do it for their advantage, deceiving others in this way.

In fact, since the phenomenon of the raw milk caught on, a "cold war" between industry and dairy farmers was touched off. Raw milk was violently attacked by the media that discredited it, but they also railed against the producers themselves. All this happens, as it is well known, when we touch the interests of large groups. Even if the information is on the side of the industry, the truth is on the side of the producers.

Raw milk is safe. Furthermore, it plays a purifying function. And it is very hygienic. The foreign bacteria that could develop are harmless and do not alter the quality because milk does not deteriorate. At maximum, it can sour. The souring is due to lactic acid, so we need not be afraid to drink it if it is no longer fresh. Raw milk still acts as a purifying factor and does not lose any of its healthful properties.

Raw milk not only keeps all its properties, but it purifies the intestinal residues and other pathogens too, while boiled or pasteurized milk goes bad. The latter is dead and no longer has any power of purification and healing. Many people buy lactic ferments in pharmacies, not knowing that raw milk is already rich in these enzymes.

So raw milk is a risk, but only for the food industry because it can decrease their profits.

EVERYONE CAN DRINK IT

Personally, I drink raw milk every day. Why do I do this? Because it is a pleasant and agreeable food, good and easy to digest, as well as one of the least expensive.

In our family, breakfast consists of a bowl of raw milk with different types of cereal, seeds, and dried fruits, or a milkshake with banana, honey, carrots, and oranges. My daughters, who are 15 and 17 years old, have drunk raw milk since they were seven months old. So far they have not had any of the childhood diseases and have grown up very healthy.

In the same way, I have been drinking raw milk for a very long time now, and my father too. My father, for example, has never taken a pill and has never received an injection since he was born. He has never had any illness; neither has he been hospitalized.

I often hear people saying, "I am intolerant to milk and cannot digest it." But I wonder how many of these persons have ever drunk raw milk. Perhaps none of them. I bet that many people do not even know how fresh milk tastes. If someone is intolerant, it is precisely because he has drunk pasteurized or boiled milk. It is obvious that not everyone can tolerate the deadly and harmful substances contained in it.

A European study carried out on 14,893 children of ages between five and 13, living in rural areas of Austria, Germany, Netherlands, Sweden, and Switzerland, showed that the consumption of raw milk is associated with a reduction of asthma (-26 percent), hay fever (-33 percent) and food allergies (-58 percent).[79]

The following are just two examples that I consider instructive; they tell the stories of two mothers:

79 Waser, M., Michels, K. B., et al, "Inverse Association of Farm Milk Consumption with Asthma and Allergy in Rural and Suburban Populations across Europe" *Clinical and Experimental Allergy*, Volume 37, Issue 5, May 2007, 661–670.

"I am a 27-year-old mother, a resident of Ospitaletto, Italy. I have two children, Andrew and George, 17 and six months old respectively. Both were born prematurely and were hospitalized for a short time for respiratory problems in the neonatal intensive care unit at the Ospedale Civile of Brescia.

"I nursed my first child with infant formula since the first days of his life, and every meal was followed by vomiting. So when he was four months old, I was forced to watch him for at least one hour after each meal in order to avoid too much vomiting. When he was six months of age, I started to give him fresh pasteurized milk, with which I noticed some improvement. However, the meals were inexorably followed by regurgitation as well as vomiting, despite not exceeding 150 cc of milk during every meal.

"The problem was finally solved in mid-December 2006, when in Ospitaletto there was installed a raw milk vending machine of the Noli company and from which one day I decided to take the raw milk for my son. From that day, Andrea gladly eats up to 200 cc at every meal and digests it completely without any regurgitation!

"With my second child, unfortunately, I had to face even more problems. I changed to five different types of infant formula. Nevertheless, Giorgio had growth problems as well as vomiting and digestion difficulty, which also caused him stomach pain. A few days before he was five months old, I tried to give him raw milk too. Again, I solved the problem!

"I talked about my case with the pediatrician, who fully supported me. Moreover, he advised me to mix in a bottle, if necessary, 30 cc of water in addition to milk, but only for my youngest child."

The second story is interesting as well:

"I am writing to tell you my story with raw milk. I went to receive allergy tests as I have done every year because I suffer from pollen allergy. Sometime before going to the out-patient clinic, from the hospital I was told to bring some products, including milk. Obviously, I brought raw milk, since I normally drink raw milk. The tests were carried out in groups of five people at a time, and everyone had brought a little milk. Of course, theirs was pasteurized milk or even worse, the UHT. By chance, for the test, allergists used the raw milk I brought.

"The result was the following: in the group of five people, three were known to be intolerant or allergic to milk for some years, but to the astonishment of the same allergists, as well as of the persons in question, they were no longer allergic!

"I explained to them that they did the test using raw milk, but most of the doctors did not want to believe it. So they repeated the test with pasteurized milk. The result: the three people still showed obvious signs of the allergy. I went out from the out-patient clinic very happy, and I also had to accompany one of these people to the nearest distributor of raw milk.

"I do not know the scientific meaning of all this, but the result seemed to me eloquent and irrefutable: Raw milk is very good for health, pasteurized milk is not!"

THE MISINFORMATION

Being updated all the time on anything and everything is not sufficient. We should also pay attention to those who distort the information, the so-called misinformers. They are people with no knowledge, sensitivity, or morality. Their purpose is to distract people from logical reasoning, staging squabbles and clinging to worthless quibbles. Their intention is to conceal facts that are bluntly real and self-evident.

Typically, they are well-trained professionals, and they are very dangerous. They are on the payroll of the government or a corporation. They are wolves in sheep's clothing. Unfortunately, they can be recognized only by very informed persons.

People who fall into their ruthless traps pay a great cost for that error either with their money or with their health, to the extent of putting their own lives in danger.

Therefore, the misinformers are scoundrels, who for a little or a lot of money are willing to sell out their fellow man. We can find them in every area of life, including when discussing the topic of milk.

In general, there are three groups saying "no" to raw milk:

1. *The misinformers.* They are funded by the industries. They maintain that raw milk is not safe or that it is even harmful to our health. According to them, we should drink only pasteurized or boiled milk.

2. *The group of the "ignorants."* They take as valid the first information that reaches their ears, and most of the time remain faithful to that information for life. They are the preferred prey of misinformers because once contaminated,

an ignorant person will infect others. It is like igniting a fire; once ignited, it burns by itself.

3. *Radical animal-rights activists.* These people, unlike the first two groups, do not admit either raw or pasteurized milk because they are against the suffering endured by animals in the cosmetics, pharmaceutical, and food industries. In order to defend the animals, they are willing to write lies about raw milk and eggs.

In the case of radical animal-rights activists, the truth lies somewhere in between. They have a point, but there is no need to exaggerate either from one side or from the other. If raw milk is good, let's just say so, and if the cows are mistreated, let's say so as well. But please, do not confuse the two things.

I believe without a doubt that animal life can and should improve. I think that the cows will have more chances to be treated better, mainly due to higher gains from the sale of raw milk.

As for the mystification of the information, baseless statements appear every year. For example, in a work by Holzer Sommers we read that the consumption of raw milk will cause children to become ill of aphtha, measles, chickenpox, and scarlet fever.

My girls are an example of the groundlessness of such statements. The facts show the opposite: raw milk cures because it immobilizes the acids. In addition, for convalescents it is a food much easier to digest.

Sommers' theory is also groundless. According to his theory, adults can no longer digest raw milk—only infants can. Also, as soon as milk comes into contact with the air, it is no longer pure, nor raw!

In the Baltic countries, people, for whom raw milk is the basic food, live more than the average age of life; this invalidates the theory of Sommers. This is further proof that the literature on raw milk is often dominated by interests other than science.

MILK DERIVATIVES

Unfortunately, almost all dairy products on the market are pasteurized, except for some cheeses. The only alternative is to buy more raw milk, of which we can use half to drink and the other half to make cheese, yogurt, cream, or butter.

To make cream, butter, or cheese, the milk must be left at room temperature for one to three days. To immediately make cheese with rennet, first bring the milk up to 36-38°C. I advise using natural rennet, which is extracted from the stomach of the lamb or calf.

On the Internet there is a lot of information about how to make yogurt or cheese. Unfortunately, many of these recipes are industrial. For this reason, we might find recipes that tell us to boil or heat the milk above 40°C. Follow the recipe but use the common sense of this book and not exceed 40°C. In fact, this is the maximum value tolerated by milk and all other types of food.

Many people do not know that whey—the liquid that separates from the curd during cheese production—does not have to be thrown away. In fact, it is one of the oldest and most natural healthy drinks. Whey was known and used since the times of the Greeks and Romans as a therapeutic and as a beauty product for bath and beauty treatments on the face.

If taken regularly, whey improves our well-being and keeps us healthy and fit. Moreover, it has a number of positive effects on organisms, and it gives the skin a bright color. It tightens the connective tissue and gets rid of annoying masses of fat. Whey is really a complete health and beauty treatment!

Another derivative of milk is ricotta. Despite being a dairy product, it cannot be defined as cheese. It is simply classified as a dairy product. It is not obtained through the coagulation of casein, but from the proteins of whey.

It is too bad that in order to produce it, the serum should be literally "re-cooked" (in Italian, "ricotto" gives the name "ricotta"). Instead of eating the ricotta, it is 10,000 times better to drink the serum, considering that at a temperature of about 100°C to which the whey is exposed to produce the ricotta, all proteins, enzymes, mineral salts, and vitamins not only become inactive, but even noxious.

Arnold de Vries, a known American researcher, in his book *The Elixir of Life*,[80] writes, "Children who have been given only pasteurized milk became ill of scurvy, rickets, digestive disorders, and other diseases in a short time."

Experiments also show that pasteurized milk and its cooked derivatives, instead of protecting us against diseases, favor them. In addition, pasteurized milk and dairy products instead of giving calcium to our bones, subtract it, causing serious problems.

---

80 De Vries, A. P., 1952. *The Elixir of Life*, USA, Chicago, IL: Chandler Book Co.

THE COLOSTRUM

Colostrum is the name given to breast milk secreted by the mammary glands during the first three to seven days after birth. It is a more yellowish and denser food than the milk which follows. Regarding milk, it is richer in protein and poorer in fat and sugar. It should be emphasized that both bovine and human colostrum are richer in immune factors than regular milk.

In the past, colostrum had a bad reputation. It was, in fact, called "defective milk" or also "witches' milk." Many doctors claimed for a long time that this particular milk should not be consumed because it would not bring any benefit to the infant. Instead, the colostrum is an essential substance for the proper nutrition of the newborn.

Apart from its immune function, colostrum plays an important role in protecting the gastrointestinal tract. In fact, it exerts an action of "coating" the gastrointestinal tract, protecting it from the entrance of foreign matter and reducing the possible sensitization of the infant to the foods that are taken from the mother.

When the mother, for various reasons, cannot provide colostrum to the newborn, it is essential to use that of colostrum donors. Children who do not get colostrum develop poorly, and when they are adults, they will have a weak immune system. Usually, they are the first to be affected by various diseases.

While children who do not consume colostrum at birth can be saved, although with all the disadvantages of the case, calves that do not drink colostrum from their mothers die. The reason is simple: while the child receives a portion of maternal antibodies through the umbilical cord, the calf cannot receive them because the strong placental barrier of the cows prevents their passage.

For this reason, the immunoglobulins in the bovine colostrum—that have a concentration 40 times higher than in human blood—are very effective against the attacks of pathogens and are great preventive and therapeutic factors.

It is interesting to observe the balancing action of colostrum on the immune system. Actually, it acts either upwards (hyperactivity), or downwards (hypoactivity). It this way, it can be used both as an adjuvant of autoimmune diseases and as a stimulant of the antibody response in case of a viral or bacterial attack. Colostrum is absolutely the most complete natural food. It is dozens of times more active than milk.

In 1981, Ballard proved the effectiveness of growth factors in the repair of damaged epithelial and connective tissue. In the bovine colostrum, these factors are about one hundred times more powerful than those found in human breast milk.

Colostrum is the only known food that contains an enzyme called telomerase, which is essential to the reconstruction of chromosomal telomeres. According to some theories, the telomeres are associated with aging by acting as a biological clock and decreasing in length as we get older.

Popular medicine has been using colostrum for the prevention and treatment of various diseases. For example, it was used as a natural antibiotic during the American Civil War. The advent of modern pharmacology has led to the dismissal of colostrum, which was later forgotten.

Colostrum is a scarce substance, given that cows give birth only once a year and the first drafts of the precious liquid are reserved for the newborn calves. Nevertheless, cows produce colostrum in an amount which is enough to enable its withdrawal for human use without depriving the calf of its share.

My parents, when our cow gave birth, used to make a kind of colostrum cake. It was a pity that the cake was baked. Apart from the cake, we always drank both colostrum and raw milk.

I do not recommend anyone taking food supplements which are made of colostrum, royal jelly, or whatever it may be. If we really want to boost our immune system or fight any disease, the best thing is to look for a farm and agree with the owner to give you some colostrum. In the stables, the cows usually give birth continuously, almost all year around.

You should not take colostrum every day, as the food supplements producers want us to believe. If this was the case, the cows would produce it the whole year. Taking it once or twice a year is more than enough to boost the immune system, but it is not fundamental if we drink raw milk regularly. Just take it on an empty stomach two to three times a day for three days.

If we really want to get the maximum benefit, for three consecutive days drink only colostrum accompanied by water. The results will be surprising. It is better to make such treatment in the spring, when the fresh grass sprouts. In addition, the cow from which we take the colostrum should eat only fresh grass.

How much colostrum should we drink? Well, ask this of a child who is just two months or a week old. What does this mean?

It means that we should not be obsessed by measuring cups or by kitchen scales. There is not a specific standard; there is not a unique dose. The scale is ourselves. Children eat as much as they want to eat, and when they are hungry. This is the rule for us too.

Consuming a determined dose means to not listen to our organism anymore. It means ignoring its signals and losing sight of its needs.

BREAST MILK

Because cow's milk is similar to that of humans, it is good that children in the first year of their life drink milk from their mother. The American Academy of Pediatrics (AAP) recommends breastfeeding at least for the first six months of life. It is even better if breastfeeding continues up to 12 months.

Breast milk is ideal for both children and for their mothers. The former are protected from infection and are less likely to develop diseases such as diabetes, obesity, and asthma, when they grow up. In the mothers, breastfeeding helps the uterus contract and quickly stop bleeding after childbirth. Breastfeeding may also reduce the risk of breast cancer and ovarian cancer, and is also a great way to strengthen the bond between mother and child.

However, starting from the sixth month of life, children can also drink raw cow's milk. I know about many mothers who have fed their babies a couple of weeks after birth with cow's milk diluted with water. When a mother does not have enough milk and cannot find a milk donor mama, the only available alternative is the raw milk of a cow, goat, or sheep.

JUANA BAUTISTA DE LA CANDELARIA RODRIGUEZ

Another interesting case of longevity is that of the Cuban grandmother Juana Bautista de la Candelaria Rodríguez.

The sprightly old lady was born on February 2, 1885, on Santa Rosa farm, in Campechuela, in the Cuban province of Granma, where she currently lives. Her date of birth is confirmed by an original document registered in Volume 1, page 35, of the registry office of the same locality cited above. Here, the child was registered 25 days after she was born, upon the declaration of her mother, Cecilia Rodríguez.

In the year of her birth, in 1885, Cuba was still a Spanish colony, the Statue of Liberty had arrived in the port of New York, and the first automobile was patented.

The super-long-living Cuban lady is the second child in a family of 13 brothers and sisters. She has survived her husband and two of her three children. Her descendants in 2012 were six grandchildren, 15 great-grandchildren and seven great-great-grandchildren.

Candulia, as her relatives and neighbors call her, said that her mother lived more than a hundred years and that her father lived "only" 96 years.

The doyenne of the Cuban long-living people, despite having lived more than half of her life without electricity and running water, says she has always been happy and content. When she was 123 years old, she said in an interview that her long life was due to the pure air of the countryside, to a healthy nutrition, and to her heart being always full of love for her fellows.

Scholars from different parts of the world often visit her in order to try to discover the secret of her longevity. Candulia's age has been scientifically demonstrated in a biomedical and psychosocial study led in 2007 by a multidisciplinary team of the Ministry of Public Health of Cuba and the Hispanic-American Center of the Third Age.

On the day of her 127th birthday, February 2, 2012, Candulia was still wearing the ring inherited from her mother in 1900, when she was 15 years old. She has told everyone she was grateful for the life she lived. And this lady is still in perfect health.

"I'm glad that life has given me this beautiful family and my country," said Candulia in an interview for the newspaper *La Demajagua*. "They say I'm the oldest woman in Cuba; I never ever imagined that. But I hope to celebrate my 130th birthday."

The Cuban grandmother has a very clear mind too. The only thing she cannot accept is the worsening of her sight, "Even if I struggle a bit to walk, the thing I am most worried about is the lowering of my eyesight, which does not let me watch TV." A geriatrician, a general physician, and a nurse take care of Juana Bautista.

Even though her age was verified by the Cuban government, the Guinness World Records does not recognize her old age. In their argumentation, Guinness authorities say that there has never been a human being who had lived more than 123 years, and that the age of 127 years of Juana Bautista de la Candelaria Rodríguez is inconceivable.

In my opinion, the Guinness World Records is either paid by some multinational pharmaceutical company in order not to exceed the already "annoying" threshold of 122 years of Madame Jeanne Calment or it suffers from chronic myopia.

HER SECRET

Candulia and her family attribute her remarkable longevity to a diet of tubers (cassava, sweet potatoes), fruits, and vegetables, and to the fact that she has never smoked or drunk alcohol or coffee. Another secret is that she never lost her enthusiasm and the will to live since she was just a little girl. The fresh air, the sun, the favorable climate, her character, and the absence of stress typical of the countryside helped do the rest.

I would not be surprised if she reaches her 130th birthday.

IS COFFEE GOOD FOR OUR HEALTH?

After water, coffee is the most popular drink in the world. Its consumption amounts to about four billion cups per day. With a world production that reached eight billion kilograms in 2010, coffee, after oil, is the second most traded commodity in the financial markets of our planet.

Thanks to its popularity, coffee has become one of the major factors of social aggregation. We drink coffee at the bar when we meet with others, at work with our colleagues, at home when we go as a guest or with our family. Today, coffee is the favorite drink of many countries. In fact, it has become part of the habits of everyone on Earth, each with their own rituals and methods of preparation.

The question arises, "Is coffee good or bad for our health?"

In order to give an objective answer to this question, we must first see where coffee is good and where it is bad. In this case, my answer will not be based on the principle "if it is good or bad," but on "where it is good or bad."

Let us see which areas are the most affected by coffee:

1. The environment
2. Producers (farmers)
3. Intermediaries (exporters, roasters, distributors, bars…)
4. Consumers

In what areas is coffee a benefit? If we think that there is more than one area, we are wrong. In fact, coffee is bad for the environment, the producers and, last but not least, the consumers. The only group which benefits form coffee is the intermediaries. Let us analyze them one by one.

THE ENVIRONMENT

The first damage caused by coffee is to the environment. What most people may not know is that the cultivation of coffee is the largest crop in the world—above the cultivation of wheat, corn, tobacco, and soy.

In the coffee plantations, pesticides, fertilizers, herbicides, and other chemicals are used without any supervision because, in the producing countries, coffee is a main resource. Laws that should regulate its cultivation and related activities are quite lax. As a consequence, there is environmental pollution, chemical poisoning, deforestation, destruction of native flora and fauna, and the risk of extinction of many animals.

276

THE PRODUCERS

Producers suffer the second harm or damage due to the coffee. Farmers who grow coffee are underpaid and reduced to slavery. According to a report presented in 2009 by the nonprofit organization ActionAid, the price paid to the farmer by the intermediary for a pound (453.59g) compared to a cup of coffee sold at the bar is one Euro cent (the net margin profit after production costs is half a euro cent). To be more precise, the net "profit" of the farmer swings from 0.2 euro cents up to 0.5 euro cents per cup of coffee.

An exemplary testimony on the exploitation of small producers in Africa comes from Uganda. *Africa* magazine interviewed Paulina Nabaaka, the owner of a farm dedicated to the cultivation of coffee. "Exporters pay us about 30 euro cents. We cannot live this way anymore. I went to a supermarket in Kampala to check how much a kilo of Nescafé costs and, to my surprise, I saw that it costs €40.70. There must be something wrong here. Why do they pay us only 30 cents and if we want to buy the same coffee we have to pay a disproportionate amount?"

Coffee does not help either the producers or the environment. As a consequence of coffee production, there is the exploitation of the labor force, occupational diseases, and violation of human rights.

THE INTERMEDIARIES

Here the music changes. Subtract one euro cent from the price we pay for a cup of coffee at the bar and the rest goes to intermediaries. For example, if at the coffee bar we pay one euro for a coffee, we know that one cent goes to the producer and the remaining 99 cents goes to the intermediaries.

But, at the end, the producer will have only half a cent of profit because the other half of the euro cent goes to cover the production costs, for example, fuel, pesticides, and other products or services that are used in the cultivation of coffee.

Some associations have also made inquiries to see who benefits in the various steps of the coffee chain. The results were nothing short of amazing. We will consider the example of the bar.

The coffee blend that the bartender buys from the roaster has a price ranging from 20 to 35 euro per kilo—depending on the quality—and a cup of coffee takes about six grams of ground coffee. Proceeding with simple arithmetic, we easily deduce that with a kilo of coffee about 166 cups of coffee can be prepared. On average, therefore, each cup of coffee costs the bartender 17 cents.

To this number we have to add 16 cents for the fixed costs of sugar, coffee machine wear, and labor force. At the end, we have a total cost of 33 cents for each cup of coffee. Through a simple calculation, we know that the profit of the manager of the bar is on average 67 cents if we consider an average price consumption of one euro, that is, income after taxes of 200 percent.

So, for every euro cent net earned by a producer, the manager earns about 134 (67 × 2) times more. But this calculation does not take into account another factor, the time. In fact, while the bartender needs a few seconds to make a cup of coffee—from which he immediately gets 67 cents of profit—it takes a year of hard work for the producer to earn his meager half-euro cent.

The total world turnover of coffee amounts to about one trillion dollars a year. Of this figure, only $10 billion is given to the poor farmers. From the 10 billion dollars, five billion dollars must be subtracted for production costs. The remaining 990 billion dollars go entirely into the pockets of the intermediaries. From a capitalistic perspective, coffee is manna from heaven because it guarantees profit maximization. As a consequence, the intermediaries do well for themselves, for the state, and for the economy, but certainly not for the producers and consumers.

THE CONSUMERS

Having addressed briefly the environmental issue and labor force exploitation in poor countries involved in the cultivation and processing of coffee, let us now try to debunk the myth that coffee cheers us up and allows us to face difficult situations.

In accordance with some surveys carried out in early 2012, there are about a billion people in the world who drink coffee. When it comes to this drink, everybody associates coffee with caffeine. However, just a few people go into the question in more depth, and no one tells us that in the coffee there is not only caffeine but there are also more than 200 other toxins. It should be pointed out as well that coffee has no nutritional value. It is nothing more than the final result of industrial processes that makes coffee anything but a healthy and nutritious product. Basically, the drink that is obtained is little more than a concentrate of aromatic elements extracted from grains carbonized at temperatures of 200-400°C.

The large-scale distribution of coffee and tea in Europe dates back to the sixteenth and seventeenth centuries. As for other agents acting on the CNS (Central Nervous System), the introduction of tea and coffee met some resistance.

In Paris, the seventeenth century proved that coffee shortens life. In the eighteenth century, German coffee drinkers risked being beaten up in case they were found consuming such a drink. Frederick II of Prussia tried to break the habit of his subjects by imposing on them a coffee fee.

In the words of Louis Lewin, a famous German pharmacologist, "Despite the many objections raised over the years against coffee and tea, the substances that act on the brain make fun of all the obstacles opposed to their spread. Their attraction grows slowly, silently, but relentlessly."

The word *silently* is perhaps the most appropriate term nowadays to describe how drugs are gradually spreading in our modern society.

In 1952, an American physician, a member of a presidential commission, defined tea and coffee drinkers as "the truest type of drug addicts."[81]

"We need a good coffee" is just a simple phrase, but it is common to summarize in a few words the strong relationship between many people and the drink. In fact, many people already know that to start driving in the morning they must first have a cup of coffee; otherwise, they will feel tired.

If these people do not drink coffee, they are not able to have a bowel movement. If they do not drink it after lunch, they fail to return to work without feeling heavy and sleepy. Many elderly people do not want to go without it because they do not want to spend the

---

81 Keller, M., September 1972, *British Journal of Addiction to Alcohol and Other Drugs*, Vol. 67, 3, 153.

day feeling groggy. The problem is that their body becomes more and more intoxicated, and the detoxification process becomes more and more slow and insufficient, making life tense rather than a source of contentment.

Newsweek magazine, in one of its investigations, defined caffeine as "a convenient drug." We already talked about how many billions of euros orbit around coffee.

Nutritionists call it "the world's most popular legal drug." The authorities that should monitor public health not only turn away from the problem and are not worried about it, but they also speculate on its gaining lots of money.

People who start their day without a cup of coffee should not be surprised if they begin to experience symptoms of fatigue, headaches, or even muscle and joint pain similar to when we have the flu. These are signs of withdrawal from caffeine, declared by Roland Griffiths, from Johns Hopkins School of Medicine in Baltimore and Laura Juliano, from American University in Washington in the *Psychopharmacology*[82] journal.

Caffeine addiction that develops in coffee drinkers, and not only in those who drink many cups a day but also in those who drink just one in the morning to wake up, is so obvious that this was inserted in the Diagnostic and Statistical Manual of Mental Disorders, the "bible" of American neurologists and psychiatrists.

Researchers have come to support this thesis after a careful review of the most influential studies on coffee and its effects on the

---

82 Juliano, L. M., Griffiths, R. R.,. "A Critical Review of Caffeine Withdrawal: Empirical Validation of Symptoms and Signs, Incidence, Severity, and Associated Features," *Psychopharmacology*, September 21, 2004, pp. 176, 1–29.

organism over the past 170 years. They chose to review the data of 57 experimental studies and nine epidemiological investigations. They found that one out of two people, including those who have skipped their appointment with the morning coffee, said they suffered from severe headaches. And 13 out of 100 people say they experience symptoms which reduce their efficiency in the workplace.

If we stop the coffee habit, the worst moments that we will face arrive 12 to 24 hours after the last cup. The symptoms depend on the daily dose to which we are accustomed. But even when drinking just a cup per day, the withdrawal symptoms peep out.

The good news is that researchers say that detoxification is simple: it is enough to gradually get used to giving up caffeine, decreasing its doses, and little by little replacing coffee with other natural drinks. The symptoms will gradually disappear, the experts say, and we will not feel the abstinence in our bodies.

To become convinced that coffee is an addictive drug, just think about the fact that no child likes its bitter taste when he tastes it for the first time. Their bodies instinctively reject it because it is a poison. Only because of their determination to join the world of adults, will they overcome this "obstacle." After that, drinking coffee as the "adults" do becomes a habit.

Many people think that coffee, when drunk with moderation, is a great energy drink, but this is only a trap! Moderate consumption of coffee is just an illusion. Sooner or later, drinking it becomes more frequent and ends up being a constant and routine habit.

"Coffee is a poison for both the body and the mind. The combination of stress and caffeine," explains Simon Crowe, a researcher at the University of Melbourne, "produces effects similar to those of a psychosis." He also affirms that coffee is a real psychoactive drug.

Coffee irritates the mucous membranes of the stomach and bladder, which then secrete mucus to defend themselves. It is the cause of poor gastrointestinal digestion and prevents proper assimilation of nutritional substances.

We should know that the bitter taste of leaves and coffee beans is due to caffeine, and it represents a defense system of the plant to avoid being eaten by insects or animals. Therefore, caffeine is an insecticide developed by the plant to paralyze or effectively kill insects that eat the coffee plant. For this reason, coffee is also one of the main destroyers of the intestinal flora, with all its consequences, and the number-one enemy of kidneys and livers.

Pregnant women should never drink coffee. Caffeine is actually a stimulant drug that easily passes through the placenta to the developing fetus and also passes into breast milk.

Recent studies have shown that coffee consumption during pregnancy increases the risk of miscarriage, birth defects, and low birth weight. Studies have also shown that coffee consumption increases the risk of sudden infant death syndrome (SIDS). Caffeine can also make it difficult for women to maintain the necessary levels of iron and calcium that are especially important during pregnancy.

It seems that coffee consumption is associated with increased levels of estrogen, which means an increased risk of breast and uterine cancer.

Why do we have a feeling of being energized when we drink coffee? Because our organism, in order to eliminate this venom, stimulates the endocrine glands, causing them to secrete hormones such as adrenaline, for example.

It is not that coffee gives us more energy. What happens is that it causes the body to use the little or much energy that is available at that moment. If we are weak and short on energy, coffee, stimulating the endocrine system, forces us to use the little energy we have. But when we feel such a surge of energy, we might think that it is due to the coffee and the sugar.

You can force a tired horse to run by whipping it, but the lashes do not give energy to the horse. They force him to use the energy he has. And if you continue whipping him, the animal will keep running until collapsing while foaming at the mouth.

Coffee is like the lash, and we will be more tired after the whipping than before. We will have less energy. And the body, to get rid of the drug, i.e., the caffeine, will use a good part of its energy.

Contrary to what hundreds of millions of people around the world think, the coffee consumed in the morning does not "wake us up," and does not get our reflexes ready. This is confirmed by a study carried out by the University of Bristol. According to the researchers, caffeine relieves withdrawal symptoms that occur during the night but does not make people more awake or alert than normal.

The study, presented at the conference of the British Nutrition Foundation, indicates that only individuals who have avoided coffee for a certain period receive a true "boost" from caffeine. "When coffee drinkers say they feel energized by the espresso or the cappuccino," say the researchers from Bristol who analyzed dozens of previous studies on the effects of caffeine, "in reality they feel better because the cup sedates the withdrawal symptoms due to the fact that during the night they did not take caffeine."

Peter Rogers, the team leader, told the BBC, "We feel a boost from caffeine because it liberates us from withdrawal symptoms. The feeling of energy occurs because we go back to normality, not because we are more dynamic than normal. If you are not a habitual consumer, you will receive a boost from the first two cups of coffee, and then you get into this cycle."

This is why after the stimulating effect—that is illusory and apparent—we are much more tired than before and have less energy, and we need other stimulants to cheer us up in a vicious, perverse, and destructive cycle!

Kidneys are among the organs that suffer because of caffeine. Their "drugged" tissues cannot hold minerals such as calcium, iron, potassium, zinc, etc., and B vitamins. Moreover, the adrenal glands, subject to overwork, deteriorate progressively.

Therefore, coffee is a real anti-food, and what is said about it, the fact that coffee is good for our health, is not true at all.

Everything the advertising says about coffee is false. We do not need to be geniuses to figure out that "the more we drink it, the more it cheers us up" is a naked lie.

Note that companies do not save money on coffee commercials, always engaging very popular and expensive celebrities and not anonymous people. The result of the advertising campaigns usually exceeds the most optimistic expectations.

Actually, there is no need to advertise coffee. Various companies just try to convince us that their coffee is better than their competitors'. The purchase is mainly based on the sympathy aroused by the testimonial, despite the fact that the different brands buy the coffee from the same suppliers and coffee roasters.

So what doctors and dieticians say is also false, that those who do not expose themselves too much simply say that when drunk "with moderation," coffee is good, helps digestion, gives a boost of energy, and so on.

Doctors who make such statements are often themselves addicted to coffee. They are acting in the same way as their colleagues in the past who were used to smoking and suggested to their patients that they smoke a few cigarettes to help them relax a little.

A good part of the world is used to cultivate coffee, cocoa, tea, sugar cane, sugar beets, and wine grapes, in order to obtain substances that are not food but stimulants—soft legal drugs. Instead, if fruits and vegetables were grown, there would be less hunger in the world and the population would certainly be healthier.

Why then all these lies about coffee? In this world, which is more and more aberrant, where ethical and moral values are disappearing, you have to follow the thread of money to find out the reason for the persistence of false theories and harmful habits.

Coffee damages to our health:

- ✓ increases stress;
- ✓ increases the loss of bone density (osteoporosis);
- ✓ impedes the absorption of essential vitamins and minerals;
- ✓ irritates stomach lining (digestive disorders);

- ✓ can cause low birth weight, birth defects, premature births, miscarriages and even infertility;
- ✓ the liver of infants cannot metabolize caffeine;
- ✓ involves the compression of blood vessels so the heart pumps harder and blood pressure increases;
- ✓ is rich in pesticides (there is no control on the amount of pesticides used);
- ✓ increases the risk of cancer in the stomach, pancreas. and lungs;
- ✓ is harmful to the nervous system;
- ✓ causes palpitations, hot flashes, anxiety, tremor, and even nervous breakdowns;
- ✓ concentration and memory loss;
- ✓ is bad for the urinary tract;
- ✓ is bad even if it is decaffeinated;
- ✓ facilitates the occurrence of cavities and yellowing of the teeth;
- ✓ ages the skin (causing wrinkles);
- ✓ creates dependency (it is a drug).

In a nutshell, coffee wears out the body because instead of increasing its strength, coffee gives a false sense of power that requires greater effort and, as demonstrated in numerous experiments, it creates dangerous cellular changes. According to a Russian study, in order for coffee not to be harmful, you should not drink more than one cup every three days. That is, no more than two cups of coffee per week at intervals of three days.

The alternative? Herbal teas, but we will talk about them in the next volume.

CHAPTER 9

REFINED SUGAR

A bee alone is better than an army of wasps.
Proverb

The majority of people, especially children, are greedy and eat sweets often. Doctors, and nutritionists in particular, have always said to us that "the brain needs sugar" or "sugars are an excellent source of energy."

Lately, however, those same doctors have begun to warn us about the dangers of sugar for our health. Are sugars our friends or our enemies?

To answer this and other questions, it is first necessary to make something clear. It is true that sugars are an important staple food in our diet because they represent the primary source for the production of the energy necessary to make our body work. But watch out. This is true only about natural sugars that have not undergone any industrial treatment.

The problem is that the majority of people identify sugar as white table sugar, i.e., "sucrose." The term "sugar" is used either in everyday language to indicate sucrose or as a broader term that encompasses all types of sugars.

Actually, there are many types of sugars. The sweetest is fructose, found in fruits and honey. Then we have sucrose (the main component of sugar cane and sugar beet), glucose (present in honey, fruits, and some vegetables), maltose (in the shoots of cereals), lactose (in milk), and many others.

Together with starch, sugars are part of the family of carbohydrates, which are an important source of energy.

GOOD AND BAD SUGARS

In addition to good natural sugars there are bad sugars, namely the industrial refined sugar such as sugar cane, beet sugar, and all the artificial sweeteners. The latter are real poisons. The fact is that white sugar, which we introduce every day into our bodies through sweets, drinks, and so on, is the product of a long industrial processing that removes all vital substances present in the beet or sugar cane. That is the starting point for producing sugar.

In a recent study published in *Nature* magazine,[83] researchers at the University of California stated that industrial sugar and other artificial sweeteners are so toxic to the human body that governments worldwide should subject them to strict laws such as those on alcohol.

Experts have suggested introducing a tax on foods and drinks that include added sugars, prohibiting their sale close to schools

83 Lustig, R. H., Schmidt, L. A., & Brindis, C. D., "Public health: The Toxic Truth About Sugar," *Nature 482*, 02 February 2012, pp. 27–29.

and setting age limits on the ability to buy them. The researchers cite numerous studies and statistics to support the fact that sugar is harmful to society in the same way as alcohol and tobacco.

Why is white sugar an unnatural substance with toxic characteristics? In the book *Dance with the Devil*,[84] G. Schwab says, "Sugar juice, from the first stage of processing the beet or sugar cane, is subject to complex industrial change: first, it is subject to purification with lime milk, which causes the loss and destruction of organic substances, proteins, enzymes, and mineral salts. Then, to remove the excess lime, the sugar juice is treated with carbon dioxide. The product then undergoes a further treatment with poisonous sulphurous acid to remove the dark color. After that, it is subject to cooking, cooling, crystallization, and centrifugation.

"In this way, we get to the raw sugar. From this point we move to the second stage of processing: the sugar is filtered and decolorized with animal charcoal. Then, to eliminate the last yellowish reflections, it is colored with ultramarine blue dye or with the blue indanthrene—deriving from tar and, therefore, a carcinogen. The final product is a white crystalline substance that has nothing to do with the rich sweet juice at the beginning of the process. This product is sold to the public to sweeten (to poison) much of what we eat."

DEAD MATTER

The American doctor W.C. Martin classified refined sugar as a poison because it has been deprived of vital principles, vitamins, and minerals. "What remains consists of pure refined carbohydrates. The

84 Schwab, G., 1963, *Dance with the Devil*. A Dramatic Encounter, UK, London: Geoffrey Bles.

body cannot use these refined starches and carbohydrates unless the proteins, vitamins, and minerals removed are present. Nature supplies these elements in each plant in enough quantities to metabolize carbohydrates of the plant in question."[85]

Naturopaths have never looked favorably at refined sugar. It is an unnatural substance among the most toxic ones on the market. The white powder obtained is completely sterile and dead. To be assimilated and digested, white sugar steals the vitamins and minerals from our bodies—especially calcium and chromium—in order at least partially to restore the harmony of elements destroyed by refining.

The consequences of this digestive process are the loss of calcium in teeth and bones, resulting in skeleton and teeth weakening. This favors the appearance of bone diseases—arthritis, osteoarthritis, osteoporosis, etc.—and tooth decay that troubles most of Western civilization.

Recent research conducted by Bart Hoebel of Princeton Neuroscience Institute found that sugar also creates a real addiction and withdrawal symptoms similar to those caused by other drugs.

Specialists argue that when we consume sugar, neurochemical changes take place in our brain that increase dopamine. This is the reason why, when we are suddenly deprived of our daily sugar dose, a real abstinence crisis is created. It is caused by the rapid absorption of sugar in the blood, which raises blood sugar and forces the pancreas to secrete insulin. The insulin hormone causes a sudden drop of blood sugar—malaise, sweating, irritability, weakness—creating the need to eat more sugar in order to feel better.

85 Martin, W. C., "When Is a Food a Food—and When a Poison?" *Michigan Organic News*, March 1957, p. 3.

SUGAR SHORTENS LIFESPAN

Another American scientific study, dated 2009, found that sugar shortens lifespan by 20 percent.[86] Researchers at the University of San Francisco added small amounts of glucose—i.e., the form taken by sugar once metabolized—into the nutrition of the worm *Caenorhabditis elegans*, which has in common with man certain genes that control longevity. The result was that the animals died before their normal lifespan was lived out.

But this is not all. The German biologist Otto Heinrich Warburg was awarded the Nobel Prize for Medicine for discovering that the metabolism of malignant tumors depends largely on their consumption of glucose. In other words, sugar is the fuel of tumors.

Refined sugar is very harmful to humans because it provides only what nutrition experts call "empty" or "naked" calories. As we just saw, it lacks all the nutrients naturally present in sugar beet and sugar cane. And if that is not enough, sugar deprives the body of valuable vitamins and minerals.

LET THE PARTY BEGIN

The sugar taken every day produces a condition of continued hyperacidity. In an attempt to rectify the imbalance, the depths of the organism require more and more minerals.

If we do a blood-sugar test immediately after the ingestion of a large amount of sugar, we will note that the pancreatic glands, being

---

86 Lee, S. J., Murphy, C. T., and Kenyon, C, "Glucose Shortens the Life Span of C. Elegans by Downregulating DAF-16/FOXO Activity and Aquaporin Gene Expression," *Cell Metabolism*, Volume 10, Issue 5, November 4, 2009, pp. 379–391.

intensely stimulated, secrete too much insulin. That leads implicitly to a lowering in blood sugar levels below the tolerated average and, hence, a state of great fatigue.

The human body—each system, organ, and tissue respectively—over a certain period of time bears all these troubles that can be more or less serious and tries to cope with them. Nevertheless, at some point nature cruelly takes revenge for all that has been done against it.

Excess sugar harms every organ of the body. Initially, sugar is stored in the liver in the form of glucose (glycogen). Since its capacity is limited, a daily intake of refined sugar makes the liver swell up like a balloon very soon. And when it is full to the limit of its possibilities, the excess glycogen goes back into the blood in the form of fatty acids that are transported to all parts of the body and stored in the less active areas—the abdomen, buttocks, chest, and thighs.

When these relatively harmless areas are fully saturated, fatty acids are then distributed in the active organs, such as the heart and kidneys, which begin to slow down their activity. Their tissues eventually degenerate and turn into fat.

The entire body is affected by a reduced ability of its organs and abnormal blood pressure is created. The parasympathetic nervous system is damaged and all the organs controlled by it, such as the cerebellum, become inactive or even paralyzed. The circulatory and lymphatic systems are invaded and the characteristics of red blood cells begin to change. After an overabundance of white blood cells occurs, the formation of tissues slows down and tolerance, together with the immune ability of our body, becomes limited so we cannot react to relatively critical situations—whether the weather is cold or warm, or whether there are mosquitoes or microbes.

Sugar consumed in large quantities gives a feeling of satiety due to the high number of calories that it contains. But where are the vitamins, the enzymes, and the minerals? Refined white sugar no longer contains any of these substances. Therefore, it does not introduce into our body any type of help for digestion. Consequently, sugar causes more damage than benefits to our health.

The body is deprived of some of its important elements and is now obligated to subtract those which are necessary for the nutrition of glands, nerves, and blood. The problems and disorders caused by refined sugar reduce the willingness to do things and affect memory. It contributes to impotence, tooth diseases, arthritis, neurosis, madness, and even suicide. Ultimately, sugar can cause any disease, including cancer. The natural food supporters maintain that for our health refined sugar is even more harmful than alcohol.

The damages of the white sweet poison are numerous and occur at all levels. For example at the circulatory level there is an increase of cholesterol and damage to the arteries, liver, pancreas (because the organ that manages the sugar level is the pancreas), weight gain and obesity, and skin problems.

It is inconceivable that governments grant sugar a preferential regime and lower its price instead of increasing it. They should give an explanation to the people about its harmful effects and the damage it causes to health. Why do doctors not say a word about this reality, and why do dentists speak so little of the dangers of sweets?

There are many studies indicating that myocardial infarction is the result of a prolonged consumption of sugar—in whatever artificial form it is—bread (both white and whole grain), and pastries. Recall that not even cooked fruit is healthy.

Replacing white sugar with virgin honey could prevent almost all of these diseases.

BROWN SUGAR

Brown sugar cane or brown beet sugar is an illusion. As explained earlier, the only thing that is brown in these sugars is their name. As explained earlier, first, sugar undergoes a type of treatment with lime milk (yes, I am talking about the material that is usually used in construction!) resulting in the loss and destruction of organic substances, proteins, enzymes, and mineral salts. After that, in order to remove the excess lime the sweet juice is treated with carbon dioxide. The product then undergoes another treatment with the poisonous sulphurous acid to remove the dark color. Then it is subsequently subject to cooking, cooling, crystallization, and centrifugation. At the end of this process we obtain raw sugar. Therefore, brown sugar will have more impurities. There is also someone who decided to lightly toast white sugar in order to give it a golden brown color to make it look like real brown sugar.

Raw or brown sugar is just a type of sugar with more impurities, which does not give it a higher nutritional value. Even if those few minerals introduced in raw or brown sugars were still organic—we saw that with cooking, organic salts become inorganic and therefore unusable—they would however be only a drop in the sea of our body's requirements of mineral nutrients.

In addition, the high price of raw sugar is unjustified. Although its production costs are lower than those of white sugar, it costs more.

THE WHITE CIVILIZATION

It has been widely demonstrated that populations not reached by the so-called "white civilization" are not subject to dental decay or any other tooth disease. With the arrival of white people and their refined foods such as sugar, sweets, alcohol, and bread, the natives of Australia, the Maori of New Zealand, the Indians of Peru and the Amazon, the red Indians of North America, and so forth, began to be subject to the same diseases as white people. So they started to queue in the dental and medical clinics of their civilization. The incidence of cavities, a disease that previously was completely unknown, began to affect the individuals in these populations until 100 percent of them were affected.

The problem today is that white sugar is everywhere. It is in bread, sausages, preservatives, and cigarettes, not to mention sweets, candies, chocolate and, of course, its use in tea or coffee. To give an example, one can of a sparkling soft drink—Coke, orange soda, etc.,—contains on average 10 teaspoons of sugar.

In the U.S., the growth in the consumption of sugar in the last 300 years is astonishing:

- In 1700, the annual per capita consumption of sugar was 1.8 kg
- In 1800, the annual per capita consumption was about 8 kg
- In 1900, the annual per capita consumption had risen to 40 kg
- In 2009, 50 percent of Americans consumed on average more than 80 kg of sugar per year.

From the late nineteenth century to the present, cases of diabetes increased from three cases per 100,000 people to 8,000 cases per 100,000 people. Since then, the percentage of obese people has increased from 3.4 percent to 32 percent. To these figures we should also add 33 percent of overweight people.

Our genetic makeup has grown in a nutritional context. From the Paleolithic Era when only 2 kg of sugar was consumed per capita each year in the form of honey, we switched to 8 kg of sugar in the nineteenth century, to then reach 70 kg at the end of the last century!

Nowadays, sugar is not only present in sweet and fizzy drinks, as we are used to thinking, but in almost all processed, transformed, and packaged foods. It is also found in hamburgers, hot dogs, sauces like ketchup, mustard, and Worcester, in many types of bread, canned or precooked foods, and so on. Today, more than 60 percent of the sugars we eat are hidden in processed foods.

A LITTLE BIT OF HISTORY

In ancient times, mankind did not even suspect the existence of sugar. Actually, in ancient Greece the word "sugar" did not even exist.

When Alexander the Great arrived in India in 325 BC, he reported that he had tasted "a sort of honey, which is located in the reeds." Three centuries later, the famous writer and Roman chronicler Pliny the Elder kept calling it *reed honey*. The word *saccharum* was born during the reign of Nero, in an era of debauchery and excess.

The increasing dose of sugar per capita in the course of history has been accompanied by many unpleasant phenomena, such as the increase of diseases, the weakening of the immune system, and the decline of entire generations. For example, the German scholar and physician of the sixteenth century Rauwolf believed that the Turks and Moors had ceased to be brave warriors after they started using sugar, roughly starting from the seventh century. Europe learned of this sweet substance that is obtained from the Indian cane at the time of the Crusades.

THE PARADOX

In East Africa, there is a tribe that eats high-fat foods such as meat and butter, but no sugar. It would be natural to think that their blood vessels are full of cholesterol, that they are affected by various coronary heart diseases, and that the destiny of this poor tribe is extinction. But actually, they do not suffer from any of these diseases at all. They do not even have dental cavities.

The inhabitants of St. Helena, instead, who like to eat a lot of sugar and very little fat, often die of a heart attack.

OTHER SWEETENERS

Fructose syrup, the name of one sweetener, relates to the image of its counterpart sugar derived from beneficial fruit, but it is actually made from corn by a process that eliminates any nutrients such as vitamins, enzymes, minerals, and all phytonutrients capable of reducing adverse metabolic effects. Fructose syrup is used in the production of sparkling beverages, fruit juices, and many industrial products and dietary preparations.

Artificial sweeteners have names such as saccharin, aspartame, and other artificial sweetening products often advertised with enticing commercial names. They are considered to be sugar substitutes and are addressed to diabetics or those who need to reduce body weight or do not want to gain fat.

Aspartame is the most famous and at the same time the most controversial synthetic sweetener. Its sweetening power is 200 times greater than that of common sugar. This substance does not exert metabolic effects on blood sugar, so people with diabetes make large use of it. Aspartame is found in thousands of foods, as well as in the so-called "light" products. Soft drinks, candy, chewing gum, and drugs contain it as well.

Nevertheless, aspartame is considered unhealthy. As a matter of fact, much research has shown its carcinogenicity in animals. In addition, many scientific studies have shown that aspartame is a threat to human health, even more dangerous than the industrial fructose. It is associated with birth defects, cancer (mainly brain cancers), increased body weight, Alzheimer's, and many other diseases.

Saccharin is a widely known substance. Our body does not metabolize saccharin and it does not provide calories to us. Its sweetening power is 500 times higher than common sugar, while its taste is quite bitter. Saccharin, like aspartame, does not increase blood sugar levels. This is why diabetics also use it.

This sweetener is contraindicated during pregnancy, lactation, and in the first three years of life. Some studies have recently shown that the sweetener is a risk factor for cancer that affects different organs of the body. It can also cause allergic reactions, hives, diarrhea, shortness of breath, tachycardia, etc.

Acesulfame K (Ace K) is another synthetic sweetener widely used in food for diabetics, in sparkling beverages, and in oral hygiene products. Its sweetening power is 200 times greater than common sugar. It can cause headaches, depression, nausea, and mental confusion, as well as eye, liver, and kidney disturbances.

There are also other synthetic sweeteners, but we are not going to analyze them. However, without being too specific, all artificial sweeteners should be totally avoided because they are all chemically synthesized and have no nutritional value at all.

WHAT CAN WE DO?

It is clear, and there is no doubt, that to remove the risk of diseases such as diabetes, heart disease, cancer, as well as many other health problems, it is necessary to adopt a healthy lifestyle where the elimination of industrial sugar and artificial sweeteners becomes a habit.

We should bear in mind that refined sugar and food preparations containing it make our body addicted to it. Therefore, if we want to eliminate sugar, we cannot do it out of the blue without suffering from violent withdrawal symptoms.

While all foods and drinks containing sucrose are harmful and acidify our body, the natural sugar fructose is more suitable to man because it has an alkalizing effect that contributes to the maintenance of good health.

Of course, only fructose contained in fresh or dried fruit has a beneficial effect. That white powder that is sold as fructose in health food stores is to be avoided, together with sucrose. In fact, it is certainly not the true fructose that you get eating good ripe, seasonal, and organic fruit.

Dried fruits such as figs, raisins, and dates are also very useful and have valid purifying effects. It is important, however, that these fruits have a biological origin because in the dried fruit of industrial preparation, sulfur dioxide, which is a poison used as a preservative, is always present and cancels all the beneficial effects of food. For those foods that require more sweetening, we can easily replace sugar with honey or grape juice or fresh apple juice.

Do not be afraid of getting fat by eating fruit. On the contrary, you should and must eat fruit whenever you feel the need for something sweet. When our body is healthy because it is well fed, it knows how to eliminate calories and anything else that is unnecessary. In fact, often the stimulus of the appetite decreases gradually when we switch to healthy and beneficial nutrition.

For school lunches, we can give our children some fruit instead of the industrial snacks. Fruit is a source of energy, vitamins, minerals, and enzymes, and also our organism absorbs it more gradually.

Remember that reading labels carefully every time we buy something is no longer useful nowadays, since 99 percent of processed foods on the market are full of preservatives, artificial sugars, and dyes. So the best choice is to buy everything fresh: fruits, vegetables, seeds, grains, milk, nuts, eggs, and so on, and prepare everything in the house.

While in industrialized countries this seems like an enterprise, in poor countries it is a normal thing. In fact, in many poor regions people are forced to buy only raw foods, such as vegetables and fruits, because they cost less, or to cultivate them directly in their own gardens.

Some dangers associated with the consumption of refined sugars:

- weakening of the immune system;
- asthma exacerbation;
- body acidification;
- heart disease, diabetes;
- gallstones, hypertension, and arthritis;
- some types of cancer;
- liver weighting (with the risk of serious diseases with damages similar to those due to alcohol abuse);
- deceiving the hunger stimulus and satiety-control system;
- reducing the elasticity of capillary walls;
- causing overweight and obesity;
- causing memory impairment;
- causing depression, irritability, anxiety, attention deficit;
- disrupting the balance of minerals;
- destruction of the intestinal flora;
- the possible development of food allergies;
- the possible weakening of the DNA structure;
- causing Parkinson's disease and Alzheimer's disease;
- causing osteoporosis;
- causing premature aging;
- reducing life expectancy.

HONEY

Honey has been collected for at least 6,000 years. Since ancient times, it was used to treat digestive disorders and to create ointments for wounds and injuries. The Sumerians used it in creams along with clay, water, and cedar oil. The Babylonians used it for cooking; the Greeks and Romans had the intuition to transfer the honey from the table to medical science and used it as a therapeutic polyvalent remedy and as a beauty product, as well as an indispensable ingredient in the kitchen.

Honey is good for children because it promotes the physiological secretion of mucus at the upper respiratory tract level. Three thousand years ago, ayurvedic medicine considered honey to have cleansing, aphrodisiac, refreshing, antitoxic, cooling, and stomach healing properties. For each specific case, there was a different type of honey: vegetable, fruit, grain, or flower honey.

Ninety-five percent of honey contains fructose and glucose, and the other part contains vitamin C, minerals, and no fat. During the production process it does not undergo any human manipulation, and for this reason honey brings many benefits to our bodies.

Honey is the only real sweetener that nature has put at our disposal. Comparing the same amount of honey to white sugar, the former provides fewer calories. In fact, 100 grams of honey provide 320 calories versus the 400 calories of a similar amount of sucrose.

Honey consists mostly of simple sugars—glucose and fructose—and thus it is easy to digest. Glucose can directly enter the bloodstream and is useful immediately, while fructose is consumed more slowly, ensuring energy spread out over time. This is why honey is recommended to be part of the athlete's nutrition, as well as the geriatric's and student's diet.

Another prerogative of honey is to have a high sweetening power, greater than that of sucrose, and therefore allowing at a dietary level little caloric deposit.

Thus, honey is a rich product with curative and therapeutic properties, and it is especially nutritional. It also has antibacterial properties, which is why it never goes bad.

Using honey to soothe a sore throat and cough is a widespread habit even among very different peoples and cultures. But are the nutrients of this thick and sticky substance really effective to fight the most bothersome symptoms of throat infection?

A group of scientists from Pennsylvania State University tried to answer this question by trying to measure the actual effectiveness of honey through numerous tests. From the experiments, the researchers found that some components of honey are able to kill microorganisms and to have an antioxidant effect on the tissues, including, of course, those of the throat. The surprising results of this study were recently published in the prestigious scientific journal *Archives of Pediatric and Adolescent Medicine*.

Honey is able to prevent damage in the inner structure of the cell caused by inflammation triggered as a result of a virus attack or a colony of bacteria.

During the experiments, the research team compared the effect of buckwheat honey with *dextromethorphan*, an active principle used in a wide range of medicines for coughs and sore throats. In all the tests, honey proved to be the best remedy to keep at bay the problems related to inflammation of the oral cavity.

Honey is also an excellent remedy for wounds and burns. This was highlighted in two different studies, a New Zealand study at the University of Auckland and an American study at the University of Wisconsin.

The study led by the New Zealand researcher Andrew Jull suggests spreading Manuka[87] honey on burns to reduce the healing time of the injury. "At best, you get to anticipate the healing of almost four days," explains the researcher. This is because honey reduces bacterial contamination in case of an open or infected wound.

The topical use of honey is also cheaper than taking other measures, for example using oral antibiotics or creams that are commonly used and that often have deleterious side effects for the patient.

Some beneficial properties of honey:

✓ contains vitamin E;
✓ contains phosphorus (useful for memory);
✓ contains iron;
✓ is an antimicrobial agent;
✓ cures burns and colds;
✓ cures ulcers;
✓ cures a sore throat;
✓ has beneficial effects on periodontal disease and gingivitis;
✓ is rich in antioxidants that fight ageing.

---

87 Manuka honey is considered to be particularly suitable in burn treatments due to its high antibacterial property. However, other types of honeys are more or less effective too.

SYLVESTER MAGEE

Sylvester Magee (May 29, 1841–October 15, 1971) was the last African-American slave in the United States. The story of Sylvester Magee is really extraordinary. He was born a slave in Carpet, North Carolina, in 1841. When he was 19 years old, just before the Civil War, he was sold at a slave market for a planting enterprise in Mississippi. In 1863, Magee fled and joined the Union Army, taking part in the storming of Vicksburg.

"I was 22 years old, and the only things I knew were plowing, scraping, and picking cotton. I also knew how to saw logs and do other things you normally do on a farm," he said in an interview.

He claimed to have been wounded in both Vicksburg and Champion Hill. At the end of the war, Magee returned to Marion County, Mississippi, as a free man.

In 1965, Sylvester Magee became famous nationwide because of his advanced age. On his 124th birthday, the citizens of Collins, Mississippi, organized a party with a five-tier cake with 124 candles on it. Governor Paul B. Johnson renamed that day "Sylvester Magee Day."

Many national magazines wrote about his life and his longevity, including *Time* and *Jet* magazines. Sylvester was a guest on the *Mike Douglas Show* and flew to Philadelphia, Pennsylvania, to participate in several television programs.

He was proclaimed the oldest living citizen in the United States by a life insurance company and received birthday wishes from U.S. presidents Richard Nixon and Lyndon B. Johnson.

Apart from being regarded the oldest person who ever existed in the United States, Magee was also acknowledged as the last slave and veteran of the Civil War.

When asked how he had managed to live so long, the former slave answered simply, "The Lord has been good to me."

Magee lived 130 years and was lucid until his last days. Those who knew him say that he was a very nice person. Unfortunately, we do not know that much about his family and his life.

In 2012, on the tomb of Sylvester Magee, the Marion County Historical Society and the Southern Monument Company erected a monument in his honor.

HIS SECRET

We do not know what Sylvester Magee's secret was. All we know is that he was thin, active, peaceful, optimistic, and confident. Usually, all these features are typical of long-living people. Let's see them in detail:

- *Skinny*, eating little and healthy, ageing more slowly
- *Active*, working or being active, staying young
- *Quiet*, not being worrisome, extending life
- *Optimistic*, positive thoughts, desire for life
- *Confident*, believing in the future, believing in life

As we will see in the next volume, the mind also plays a key role in the lengthening of life. Being optimistic and hopeful at first glance would seem a trivial thing, but in reality it means "to plan" and "to set" our subconscious to lengthen our lives.

We have no information about Magee's nutrition either. However, his lean physique suggests that he followed a fairly healthy diet.

MICROWAVE OVEN? NO, THANK YOU!

It is estimated that today, about 95 percent of American households have a microwave oven. This quite certainly means that people are switching from the habit of cooking with the traditional oven to the use of the revolutionary microwave. At the end, this new habit seems quite right: it is more convenient, faster, more practical, and cheaper than a traditional oven.

Its use has become so common that by now only a few people raise the question about whether or not it is bad for our health. People naively think that if everyone uses it, and no one has ever died from using it, we can trust others and use the microwave safely. But these people are wrong.

A very significant study about the risks related to food cooked in the microwave is the study of Professor Bernard Blanc of the University of Lausanne and Dr. Hans U. Hertel, an independent scientist with years of experience in the food and pharmaceutical industries.

In 1989, Blanc and Hertel suggested to the Swiss Natural Fund, together with the University of Lausanne, a research on the effects on humans of food cooked in a microwave, but it was rejected. For this reason, the research was downsized and carried out with private funds.

Eight volunteers were tested. They followed for some months the same diet, and every 15 days they were administered on an empty stomach:

5. Raw foods.
6. Food cooked by conventional methods.
7. Food thawed or cooked in the microwave.

Shortly before meals and after 15 and 120 minutes, blood tests were carried out. Note that the volunteers were not aware of the method of cooking of what they were eating and therefore psychosomatic conditioning was excluded.

The tests revealed significant differences between the effects on the blood of the food cooked in the microwave and the effects of the food cooked with conventional methods. In particular, among the effects of the former type of food, it was observed that there was a significant reduction in hemoglobin and an increase in hematocrit, leucocytes, and cholesterol. Moreover, there were alterations in the cell membranes.

In the reports of this study it was written, "The foods cooked in a microwave oven, as compared with the non-irradiated ones, cause in the blood of the examined people alterations that indicate the beginning of a pathological process, just as in the case of a cancerous process at an early stage."

Also registered was the passage by induction of the microwave energy from processed foods to the human body by resorting to bioluminescence.

Rarely has research provoked a similar storm. Professor Blanc disassociated himself quite immediately from the conclusions of the study, fearing for the safety of his family as well as for his workplace.

Shortly after, the FEA, the association of appliance retailers in Zurich, reported Dr. Hertel, and on March 19, 1993, the court in the Canton of Berne, forbade him to disclose his findings or he would have to pay a fine of 5,000 Swiss francs. Such a verdict was then confirmed by the Federal Court in Lausanne.

In 1998, the European Court of Human Rights in Strasbourg recognized in the above verdict a serious violation of freedom of expression and ordered a compensation of 40,000 Swiss francs, a derisory compensation if compared with the cost of the proceedings and the economic and professional damage suffered by Hertel. At that point, the Federal Court ruled that Hertel could disclose his findings but on the condition he declare them as not scientifically proven.

Since then, an inexplicable curtain of silence has fallen over the issue of microwave ovens. As always, when there are great interests at stake, the truth becomes very difficult to find, hidden as it is by great pressures that exert their influence not only on the media but also especially on the scientific world and the institutions attached to it.

Scientists who have the intellectual honesty and courage to oppose this logic can be counted on one hand, and in most cases they are threatened, denounced, vilified, and persecuted in every possible way, as evidenced by Hertel's story. At the end of this section you will find an interview with Dr. Hertel by Nicholas Bawtree.

Who discovered microwave cooking? The official version says that Percy Spencer, an employee of Raytheon, in the United States, while manufacturing magnetrons for radar equipment, discovered the possibility of cooking food with microwaves. In 1946, Raytheon patented the microwave cooking process and, in 1947, it built the first commercial oven, called Radarange. However, there is another unofficial version.

This version maintains that microwave cooking was originally developed thanks to research by some German scientists who, in order to provide logistical support during the invasion of Russia, devised an invention that would allow the preparation of a large number of meals in a short time to be supplied to troops and that would even facilitate food preparation in submarines.

After the war, the Allies discovered the documentation of the medical research performed on these devices and brought them to the U.S. for further scientific research. As a result, Raytheon made the first microwave oven commercially available in 1947.

After the Second World War, the Soviet Union experimented with microwaves, and since 1957 the Institute of Radio Technology of Klinsk, Belarus, carried out research.

After performing a thorough research on the biological effects of microwaves, the Russians declared these devices outlawed, warning the international community of the biological and environmental risks that may arise from the use of these ovens.

What follows is a short summary of the studies carried out in Russia and published by the Atlantis Raising Educational Center of Portland, Oregon.

The study states that in almost all foods tested, carcinogenic compounds were found, and that the timing of food exposure to microwaves were not greater than those necessary for the purposes chosen, i.e., cooking, thawing, or heating.

Here is a summary of some of these results:

- In heating meat, d-Nitrosodiethanolamines are formed, which are known to be carcinogenic. Moreover, a degradation of the proteins occurs as well.
- Milk and cereal transform some of their amino acids into carcinogens.
- Very short exposures of raw, cooked, or frozen vegetables, transform their alkaloids into carcinogenic compounds.
- The thawing of fruit turns the content of glycosides and galactosides into carcinogens.
- Formation of carcinogenic free radicals in vegetables, especially roots (beets, turnips, etc.).
- Decrease in the nutritional value from 60 to 90 percent in all tested food, decrease of the bioavailability of the complex of vitamin B, C, and E, and of essential minerals and lipotropic factors, the substances capable of modifying fat's metabolism.

For a better understanding of why the microwave is so harmful, we need to know how it works. But first it is necessary to make a clarification: when a polarized molecule is immersed in an electric field, it tends to orient in the direction of the electric field. If the electric field is repeatedly reversed, the molecule is forced to reposition itself in every reversal field.

After having clarified this aspect, we should know that the microwave oven operates according to the same principle. It is in fact equipped with a device called a magnetron that generates a variable electromagnetic field, namely, the microwave radiation (MW).

When we turn on a microwave oven, we saturate its compartment with radio waves of a wavelength of 12 cm at a frequency of 2.45 billion. So the molecules, especially those of water but also those of lipids and proteins, reverse their position 2.45 billion times per second without having a moment of rest in a specific field. The cells filled with water enter a giant mess and so the friction releases heat, which heats the food. The molecules and cells are polarized in a destructive manner and, as many scientists have demonstrated, all life ends. This is how free radicals are born, which are precisely those that cause severe disturbances to the organism.

Because of the immense amount of energy, the cells in the food open explosively and their biological structure dies. In the microwave, foods are subjected crucially to a strong and unnatural vibration.

The proteins are more altered than in other cooking processes. Milk fat is transformed into giant balls. Vital elements such as vitamin C or folic acid are destroyed or degraded.

During the millions of years of evolutionary history, the

human being has never come in contact with this type of nutrition that affects the body like a poison. Various detailed research papers that have shown the effects of the food cooked in the microwave have proved this.

Here are some of the stages of the undertaken studies:

1973. P. Czerski and W. M. Leach (USA) show that microwaves cause cancer in animals.

1975. Studies on broccoli and carrots cooked in a microwave detect the deformation of the molecular structure of nutrients.

1987. A German study shows that there is irreversible damage to the eye in the case of prolonged exposure.

1988. A study of the American National Council for Radiation Protection highlights that the children of women who use microwave ovens have a higher chance of birth defects.

1989. According to a study conducted in Vienna, cooking in the microwave causes significant changes in food proteins, especially in milk for infants.

1990. At the University of Leeds it is highlighted that cooking in a microwave oven is not hygienically safe.

1992. The research of Hertel and Blanc shows a significant change in the blood of people who eat food cooked in microwaves.
1993. David Bridgman, kinesiologist with many years of experience, said, "99.9 percent of my patients suffering from various forms of allergies prove to be extremely sensitive to foods cooked in a microwave."

1994. An American research shows that the habit of heating leftover food in the microwave is potentially dangerous because the uneven cooking does not guarantee protection against salmonella.

1996. A research highlights the migration of particles of PVC casings used to cover the food during microwave cooking to the food itself.

2000. The University of California detects migration by enclosures for microwave of the carcinogen substance dietilexiladepate in an amount ranging between 200 and 500 ppm (the limit of the FDA is equal to 0.05 ppm). Among the migrated substances are also identified xenoestrogens. The latter substances are related to the decrease in spermatozoos in men and to the onset of breast cancer in women.

Different research shows that when heated in microwaves, infant milk can be subject to modification of amino acids, with a consequent toxicity or alteration of the nutritional value.

Another problem of microwaved food is that its color and flavor is not as strong when compared to food cooked in the traditional way, especially in the case of foods that contain pasta. This fact has developed and encouraged the production of additives that can be used in foods for microwave and that artificially reproduce the colors and flavors that consumers expect to find.

Eating food cooked in this way produces alterations of blood, cells, and the immune system, making it more prone to a cancerous condition.

Presented as "miraculous," able to cook food quickly, ideal for those who do not have much time, the microwave is one the leading causes of diseases.

The food cooked in a microwave tastes so disgusting that food industries had to use additives, colorants, artificial flavorings, and other junk substances to reproduce as much as possible the natural flavor. Or, alternatively, they have added these substances to the packaging and, by doing so, the chemical additives go directly into the food.

Therefore, we must not be surprised if those elegant particles of "time saving," such as plastic containers that are ready to be put in the oven, end up in the food when heated up.

In a previous chapter we saw that plastic is toxic when in contact with food. Imagine if it is combined with microwave and additives. In fact, most of the containers for microwave ovens are made of plastic. Putting it all together, we create a monster food. Ignoring this aspect means to have no care for our own health.

But if this technology is so dangerous, why has no one ever said anything? The answer is that those few persons who have tried to say out loud what the problem was were immediately thwarted and silenced, as in the case of Dr. Hertel.[88]

---

88 Interview of Nicholas Bawtree to Dr. Hertel extracted from the Italian magazine *Terra Nova* published in September 2006.

INTERVIEW WITH DR. HERTEL

Dr. Hertel, why did you lose the lawsuit brought against you by the appliance retailers when the results of your studies on the dangers of food cooked in the microwave were so clear?

Hertel: It could not go otherwise, since Professor Michael Teuber of the Institute for Food Science at the Swiss Federal Institute of Technology in Zurich who, in the process of representing the official science, said that, according to research underway at his institute, foods cooked in the microwave did not represent any risk to consumers.

However, the results of that research were never published. Why?

Hertel: Simply because its conclusions were not consistent with what was stated at trial. This means that Teuber had intentionally lied to the court in the name of industry. Even in the light of the final results of that thesis, Teuber has never corrected his statement and, at present, not even the court has corrected its verdict.

Do these things happen often when scientific research goes against the interests of large economic groups?

Hertel: All the scientific research that is not in line with the interests of the industry or military sector not only is not supported but is also suppressed as much as possible. The private research that shows results that go against the interests of the powerful are vilified and persecuted in every possible way. This has been common practice for at least a century now, without the public being aware of it. Also, because people prefer trusting the authorities, especially with regard to the scientific world, and believing in the integrity of the universities and the public organizations, they are not willing to believe in the corruption of governments, industries, and, even less, of science.

What were the criticisms of your research on microwave ovens?

Hertel: The industry defined our study as not being scientific because we used only eight people and because some of the results obtained did not show significant changes but only trends included within scientifically-acceptable limits. According to the official science, tests must be repeatable to be scientifically correct, and so they need statistically significant results conducted through thousands of tests on animals. Any self-respecting scientist should arrive at the conclusion that this type of procedure is totally unacceptable since it makes no common sense.

In our experiments we did not want to endanger the volunteers who had offered to act as guinea pigs. Therefore, we submitted them to a single ingestion of food cooked in a microwave with a time of two weeks for recovering. In this context, no blood alteration could ever be "significant." A persistent tendency would give the necessary information to see in which direction these effects could be developed.

Can you explain the underlying principle that makes the microwaves so dangerous?

Hertel: The microwaves technologically generated are in contradiction with nature and are, therefore, toxic. We are talking about a type of energy based on the principle of alternating current, while the natural energies are based on pulsed DC. The sun radiates its light in a continuous manner, creating a continuous flow of pulses that are able to lead and support life on Earth. Instead, the microwaves, following the continuous reversals of polarity, create a "shaking" and separation effect that causes a decay process in biological tissues and also in inorganic tissue.

The outcome is cancer. Unfortunately, microwaves have the same effect on food and, through it, on the human body. The food molecular structures are deformed and then altered in their form and quality.

Their energy value, determined by the shape of their structure, is altered, and this process makes food toxic, while from the point of view of chemical composition the molecules are the same and can be analytically detected. For this reason, the effects of microwave cooking in a food are not evident immediately, but only in the long term as, for example, with the development of any cancer.

Even wireless communication, in the same way as short-wave transmissions and cellular telephones, work with the same microwaves regardless of their frequency. Therefore, in principle, they have the same effects as the microwave ovens. This microwave heat deforms and destroys the cells of the brain and the human body, but also those of animals and vegetables. Today we live in a huge microwave oven that is cooking slowly.

What can we do then?

Hertel: It is necessary to invest in environmentally friendly alternative technologies. This would require that science be based on natural laws instead of trying to transform the natural processes to its liking, as it is happening today. Nature communicates according to the principle of the direct current without doing any harm to anybody.

CHAPTER 10

TABLE SALT

"You are the salt of the Earth"
Jesus in the Gospel

When I was little, my grandmother often told me that her parents, in order to get a little salt, had to travel two or three days with their cart full of sacks of grain to a market where they would trade the grain for salt. It was a long, difficult, and dangerous journey.

Now times have changed. Salt is abundant and at a good price. Just walk to the nearest shop or go to the supermarket, and you'll find salt. At less than one euro, we can buy a kilo of salt. It is really cheap, isn't it? No, it is not.

There are invisible costs to using salt that are hundreds of times greater than the economic cost. When it is said that a shop is doing huge discounts on some products, people are willing to queue for hours just to buy something at a good price. Let's say that someone, after seven hours of queuing, saves €60 on a pair of shoes whose price was €200 before.

Did this person make a deal? Of course he did not. To the price of €140 (€200, at a 30 percent discount) already paid for the shoes, they must also add the price of their time. Rather than standing in the queue for seven hours, they could have chosen to work. For example, if that person had done some work at €20 per hour, in seven hours he would have earned €140 against the €60 of the discount.

Therefore, the real price of their shoes in economic terms would be:

Price of the product €200 − €60 discount + €140 potential work =

200 − 60 + 140 = €280

It is the same thing with salt. Besides the visible price we pay for the salt, we must also add its damage to health and the less time we will live because of it. I would say that it is quite a high price.

A BIT OF HISTORY

The use of cooking salt dates back to about 10,000 years to the Neolithic age, with the emergence of agriculture, which profoundly changed the lifestyle of man. The change in nutrition that came from the need to preserve food for long periods of time required the widespread use of salt. Man has always tried to preserve food as long as possible because of the fear of suffering hunger. This is why many perishable foods, such as cheese, meat, fish, and vegetables, were sprinkled with this substance.

At the beginning, salt became part of human nutrition primarily as a preservative. Only in later times, in fact, was it determined that changes in taste made salt indispensable to flavoring dishes and caused it to be used in the preparation and cooking of food.

THERE IS NO LONGER A NEED FOR SALT

The first domestic refrigerator was put on sale in 1913. Now, although more than a hundred years have passed since the need to use salt to preserve food has disappeared, people still prepare their food as if salt was important. It is the same as if we ignited a fire in our home in winter while having a great heating system.

There have been periods in history when salt was worth almost as much as gold. That was the case with my great-grandparents, who exchanged a carriage full of wheat for 10 kg of salt.

This was done for two reasons. First, there were difficulties related to its supply. Salt was not available everywhere, and those who did not have it had to buy it from other people. Second, it was the only way to preserve food, especially in summer. Throughout history, men have endured famines, many of which were due to the scarcity of salt.

In the past, the fact of not being able to preserve food for long periods of time involved an enormous expenditure of resources, but also the risk of experiencing starvation and death. Salt was a life insurance policy, and those who possessed it abundantly were considered rich men.

Note that the word "salary," of Latin origin, derives from the word salt, because in ancient times the soldiers were paid in salt. In ancient Rome, during the first century AD, centurions were paid about three kg of salt per month. The armies were in need of salt either as a bargaining chip or as a disinfectant. Just to give some examples: one kilo of bread at that time cost about the equivalence of €3 in our day; one liter of wine cost €12; one gram of gold cost €4; and one kilo of salt cost €375. This means that with 10 kg of salt someone could buy one kg of gold.

Salt was so valuable, not for its taste, as many mistakenly think, but for its anti-bacterial and food-preservation properties. In the Bible, we find salt being used in many metaphors or parables as a symbol of wisdom, immortality, and eternal covenant between God and man. In the Gospels, Jesus exhorted his disciples to be the salt of the Earth, that is, to be a force capable of preserving humanity from the results of sin.

NOT ALL SALT IS BAD

I have not used cooking salts or table salts since 1988 when I was 14 years old. I only eat meals prepared at home, so it is impossible that there is salt hidden in processed food. I eat only fruits, vegetables, milk, fresh eggs, sprouts, seeds, nuts, and other types of foods, all of them completely raw.

Therefore, does it mean that for all these years I have never taken salt? Of course I have. I have eaten salt every day. Otherwise I would be really ill, as my sister was years ago.

The fact is that all the salt that we need for our health, including the sodium found in kitchen salt, is found in sufficient quantities in natural products such as fruits, vegetables, grains, milk, and eggs. But that's not all. These salts, unlike the industrial ones or those artificially produced by man, are organic. Sea salt is not organic.

Many people mistakenly believe that sea salt was formed over millions of years by the sediments of living organisms. This is true, but only in part. Saying that organic sediments form salt is like saying that the sun illuminates the universe. It lights the universe, but how much?

This statement is overestimated and very exaggerated. In fact, in the composition of refined salt, these sediments represent less than 0.1 percent. That is, in one kg of salt there is less than one gram of the former organic salt.

Why former organic? Because even salt dies along with the algae or fish to which it belongs. Only living plants have the ability to transform—and preserve—dead salt to living salt. This is possible thanks to the photosynthesis of the plant. Therefore, salt is good as long as it remains organically bound to the enzymes and vitamins of the plant. After that, it reverts to what it was before, a dead salt which is an inactive element.

Where does salt come from? It comes from the rocks. For more than 4.5 billion years, the weather, the rivers, the volcanic activity of the oceanic crust, and the action of the seas themselves, have stolen the salts from continental rocks through slow erosion.

Therefore, it is useless to spend so much money on salt that comes from the Himalayas, maybe because it is 250 million years old and is considered pristine. That is ridiculous! What is the difference between eating a polluted inorganic substance and an unpolluted one? Or, in other words, what is the difference between eating a polluted poison and an unpolluted poison?

Once again, all salt that man needs is already contained in

living foods. Some people say that between table salt and unrefined sea salt there is a big difference in quality. Sea salt is made up of about 84 elements, while table salt has only two elements.

That is true, but if in terms of health we compare sea salt with the salt of plants, the benefits that derive from plants are millions of times greater than those that are obtained from stones. Indeed, sea salt is a rock. Would we prefer to eat plants or stones? I think I know the answer.

There is a Moldovan proverb that says, "When two dogs are fighting over a bone, a third dog comes and steals it." This is also true when it comes to salt. The three dogs are the three main types of salt: table salt, sea salt, and vegetable salt. The bone is reason. While some argue that table salt is beneficial to our health, and others say that sea salt is good, in fact reason is on the side of vegetable salt, i.e., the salt from plants.

TABLE SALT OR SEA SALT

Let us debunk a myth. Many think that table salt and sea salt are two different salts. In fact, they are both sea salts. The difference is that salt takes its name according to the processing that it undergoes.

There are two main sources of salt. The salt dissolved in waters of the seas and oceans represents the first one, which is also the larger of the two. The salt as a solid mineral in land deposits represents the second one. The latter is nothing more than residues of ancient seas or underground lakes which evaporated a million years ago. From them, one can extract the sodium chloride already in solid form called rock salt, also known as *halite*. In short, even if the sources are different, both types of salt have the same origin: the sea water. The difference, as mentioned previously, consists in the production process.

Sea salts may undergo little or no processing at all (*unrefined sea salt*), being somehow worked (*whole salt*), refined (*table salt*), or even transformed (*iodized salt, fluoride salt*, i.e., transformed with the addition of other minerals such as iodine, fluorine, iron, sodium ferrocyanide, and others). These minerals are not organically bound. Actually, they only cause damage to our bodies.

Another feature that puts salt in a bad light is that most of the time both sea salt and table salt are dried in ovens at a temperature that goes from 200 to 600 degrees. In this way, processors evaporate even the already minimal benefits of a whole sea salt.

THE DAILY REQUIREMENT

While some people eat salty foods for the simple pleasure of a savory taste, others eat salt for fear of getting ill.[89] Can we do without it? Of course we can.

There are some people who do not suffer from high blood pressure, like Eskimos and many African tribes. Studying their nutrition habits, sodium was identified as a factor responsible for this because these people do not consume any kind of salt.

In recent decades, the progressive industrialization of food and the spreading of fast-food restaurants have increased salt consumption

89 The belief that salt is an essential food for our health is widespread. Remember what my sister (a medical doctor) used to say about salt? Almost all doctors recommend its consumption. They say that it is a good thing to reduce its consumption, but not eliminate it altogether. According to them, salt is useful for its sodium content.

per capita. In many countries it has come to an average of 15–20 g per day. This is an amount 20–30 times higher than normal when we consider that our body needs only about 180–500 mg of sodium per day in order to work well. In table salt, this quantity corresponds to about 0.45–1.25 g.

But table salt and sea salt also have another problem: the chlorine. Chlorine is a poison whose concentration in table salt is so great that, with a glass of concentrated salt solution, we can take away someone's life. It is precisely the chlorine that gives to salt its preservative, disinfectant, and antibacterial properties. It is indeed a substance that suppresses life.

There is extensive literature showing that salt is responsible not only for disorders such as increased blood pressure and, therefore, cardiovascular disorders, but also it can cause kidney damage. It is involved in the onset of osteoporosis and is a major factor in the onset of stomach cancer. Suffice it to say that in the 1930s, before the spread of refrigeration, stomach cancer was the leading cause of death in Europe and Japan.

Although the use of salt seems harmless to us, that substance is one of the main problems for our health. However, for the food industry, salt is the flavor enhancer most efficient and with the lowest cost that exists.

SALT IN INDUSTRIAL FOODS

Salt that is added to foods during cooking or at the table constitutes only a fifth of our sodium consumption, namely, 20 percent of it. Another five percent comes from the sodium found naturally in foods—fruits, vegetables, nuts, milk, eggs, cereals—but more than half of the sodium we eat, at least 75 percent, comes from processed foods.

The food industry, in addition to common salt, adds to our food other sodium compounds such as the preservative sodium nitrate, the flavoring monosodium glutamate, or sodium bicarbonate, which is a leavening agent.

"Some pizzas are saltier than the Atlantic Ocean," warns the nutritionist concerned about the amount of salt we eat.

Several newspapers on health have indeed reported high levels of salt in both takeaway pizzas and in those in supermarkets. Some pizzas contained more than 10 g of salt. A simple pizza, for example the pizza Margherita, contains "only" 800 mg of sodium per 100 g. Knowing that a Magherita weighs 300 g on average, it is easy to calculate its salt content: 800 × 3 = 2,400 mg of sodium, the equivalent of 6 g of salt.

If we eat a pizza with ham, to the 2,400 mg of sodium of the simple pizza we must also add the quantity in sodium of 150 g of ham. Knowing that 100 g of ham contain 2,600 mg of sodium, we can calculate that a pizza with ham contains 2,400 + (2,600 × 1.5) = 6,300 mg of sodium, the equivalent of 15.75 g of salt! In this case, it exceeds 18 times the required daily average of sodium. And that is just for a pizza.

WAITER, I'D ALSO LIKE . . . SOME IRON POWDER

If we pay attention, doctors normally prescribe a regime without salt to people with a disease. If salt is harmful to the ill person, the same applies to a healthy person. Medicine forbids it because it has contributed to the appearance of the disease.

Only plants are able to absorb and transform the inorganic substances of the earth into organic ones. This is why plants are the intermediate step for our food.

Just as we cannot feed ourselves on stone, iron, or glass dust, we are not equipped to digest and absorb salt. The proof is that we eliminate it without its chemical structure being too changed unless, obviously, the salt has not been illegally infiltrated in the body, constituting the cause of a disease in the future.

Nitrogenous calcium and superphosphate are poisons to our body, and the same is true for table salt.

Each gram of salt contains approximately 0.4 g of sodium (400 mg). In normal conditions, our body eliminates daily from 0.1 to 0.6 g of sodium, and this quantity must be replenished with the diet but not with the addition of salt to food, since the sodium contained naturally in foods is enough to meet what our body needs.

Amount of sodium in some raw foods per 100 g of product		
Vegetables	**Fruits**	**Milk**
Artichoke – 94 mg	Coconut – 20 mg	Sour Cream – 80 mg
Celery – 80 mg	Melon – 16 mg	Whey – 54 mg
Spinach – 79 mg	Raisins – 11 mg	Milk – 49 mg
Beet – 78 mg	Papaya – 8 mg	Butter – 11 mg
Dandelion – 76 mg	Avocado – 7 mg	
Carrots – 69 mg	Pomegranate – 3 mg	**Eggs**
Parsley – 56 mg	Grapes – 2 mg	Egg white – 166 mg
Sweet potatoes – 56 mg	Strawberries – 2 mg	Egg – 130 mg*
Fennel – 52 mg	Pear – 1 mg	Egg yolk – 48 mg
Broccoli – 33 mg	Apple – 1 mg	
Cauliflower – 30 mg	Apricots – 1 mg	
Arugula – 27 mg	Pineapple – 1 mg	
Red Leaf Lettuce – 25 mg		
Cabbage – 18 mg	**Nuts**	
Red Potatoes – 18 mg	Peanuts – 18mg	
Corn – 15 mg	Pine nuts – 2 mg	
Cassava – 14 mg	Walnut – 2 mg	
Pumpkin – 7 mg	Pistachio – 1 mg	
Mushrooms – 6 mg	Almonds – 1 mg	
Potato – 6 mg		
Lettuce – 5 mg		
Tomato – 5 mg		
Onion – 4 mg		

*Some people might wonder, how is it possible that 100 g of one egg contain more sodium than its two distinct parts? This is due to the ratio of sodium that exists between egg white (70 percent) and its yolk (30 percent). In fact: $(166 \times 0.7) + (48 \times 0.3) = 130.6$ Instead: $(166 \times 0,5) + (48 \times 0,5) = 107$ < **130,6**

As we can see from the table above, fruits and nuts and grains are not very rich in sodium. Instead, vegetables, eggs, and dairy products are rich in it. Let us now see the amount of inorganic sodium in some common foods in the food industry.

Amount of sodium in some processed foods per 100 g of product	
Raw ham – 2,600 mg	Margarine – 800 mg
Pecorino – 1,800 mg	Pizza Margherita – 800 mg
Salami – 1,600 mg	Parmesan – 750 mg
French fries – 1,070 mg	Industrial bread – 300 mg
Sausage – 900 mg	

It has been found that humans are able to absorb minute amounts of inorganic substances. For example, from a tablespoon of salt our bodies absorb only a millionth of a gram. The remaining, almost everything, tarnishes the blood and organs, stimulating the proliferation of diseases or their emergence.

This reduced ability of our organs to assimilate minerals is due to the biochemical processes. The assimilation of table salt would require millions of these reactions.

Why go crazy looking for a cure when actually, in fresh foods, we have available all the nutritive salts in organic form? The amount of salt—recall that table salt is not included in the category—that man needs is found in sufficient quantities in fresh foods.

Indirect evidence can be seen in monkeys that live without salt and without all the diseases that afflict humans. Even if they were in need of salt, surely they would not use the one extracted from the mines, 300 meters deep. It would be easier for them to obtain it from the fruits they eat.

SALT SWELLS

It is known that salt causes thirst. Therefore, liquids are necessary to dilute and reduce its toxicity. After all, it is a foreign body. This causes a number of serious consequences: all tissues and artery walls are consumed, the lumen of the blood vessels is reduced, and blood pressure increases.

Our body is a complex hydraulic system. Problems start when it begins to clog. Apart from the "pipes," our hydraulic system also has a multitude of filters, such as cell membranes. When the filters—the pores of the cells—begin to become clogged, the cells no longer receive enough nourishment and oxygen, nor can they expel waste.

Moreover, to protect themselves, the cells release water to the intercellular fluid to dilute the excess of salt, and in so doing they lose elasticity and shrink. This causes a chemical imbalance of the cell, resulting in a loss of potassium.

The low levels of potassium cause, in turn, that a greater amount of sodium is able to penetrate the cell membrane. When the sodium level of the cell increases, water begins to accumulate in order to dilute it, causing the cell to swell. Over time, the continued destruction of the balance of cellular fluids can calcify, ruin and destroy muscles, valves, and coronary arteries, and may culminate in heart failure.

With the increase in body mass, also the skin acquires a spongy and sick appearance: cellulite, love handles, etc. By eliminating the consumption of salt, we eliminate not only the cosmetic damage but also we help reduce mortality from cardiovascular and cerebrovascular diseases, renal failure, and many other diseases. In the north of Japan, where diets contain more than 30 grams of salt per day, about 40 percent of the population suffers from hypertension.

The person who uses a lot of salt is often tormented by thirst and hunger.[90] Of the 15–20 grams of salt one eats regularly by nutrition, healthy kidneys can eliminate only 4–5 grams. Therefore, people who eat very salty foods sweat more than normal and cannot bear hot weather.

The body is not able to eliminate all the salts. The remaining salts are deposited everywhere, together with a number of other acids that cause numerous diseases, especially atherosclerosis. Salt destroys vitamins and enzymes.

NOT EVEN RATS LIKE IT

Dr. L.K. Dahl, from Brookhaven National Laboratory, when comparing hypertension in various populations of the world, discovered that it was common in societies where salt consumption was above average and it was almost absent in those who kept low-sodium diets. The results of his studies were confirmed as well by the observation of the effects of salt over a period of 20 years on more than 32,000 rats.[91]

To the doctor, bewilderment was even greater when, after the end of the experiment, he found that in many guinea pigs the blood pressure did not decrease anymore. So for healing, we need something more than a diet regime without salt. What can help is only a raw foods diet based

---

90 Salt causes addiction, nervousness, stress, dissatisfaction, and nervous hunger.

91 Dahl, L. K, "Salt and hypertension," *The American Journal of Clinical Nutrition*, 25(2) , February 1972, pp. 231–244.

on cereals (buds), legumes, vegetables, and fruits, all rich in enzymes.

Dr. A. Waerland writes in his book *Salt Damages your Health!*[92] that after the Second World War a soldier who was ill and dying had an overload of salt. He went to a doctor who favored natural cures. The doctor prescribed him a period of fasting. He could drink only water.

After a week, the soldier still eliminated five grams of salt through his urine. Where did it come from, since the soldier had not taken salts for quite a while? From this example we see how toxins settle in our body and cause all possible suffering. Sometimes, salt crystallizes and generates rheumatism and arthritis.

SWOLLEN ANIMALS

The excessive use of salt in human consumption has generated a similar practice in animal feed in the sense that calves are gorged on animal feed mixed with various types of inorganic salts that cannot be assimilated—a kind of chemical fertilizer.

With the help of water that builds up due to the accumulation of salt in the tissues, the animals grow fast in weight; they "swell" with water and toxins. The size normally reached by the animals in a year is now reached in just three months. It is clear that this meat will shrink in the saucepan when it is cooked. Of course, the calf would probably get sick in a few days because of this type of nutrition and eventually die.

Some people try to lose weight by eating a lot of meat. But they do not know that through the meat, they intoxicate their bodies even more.

---

92 Waerland, A., Wiberg, N., 1948, *Kochsalz schädigt ihre Gesundheit!* Schweiz, Zürich: Verl. Schweiz. Verein f. Volksgesundheit.

THE TRADITIONAL DIET

Salt, when used to the extent required by the culinary art of today, favors disease. However, there is also another aspect apart from health: flavor. With the use of salt, taste buds eventually weaken and degenerate to the point that the individual is no longer able to appreciate the delicious flavors of natural foods like fruits. People whose taste has been ruined from taking too much salt refuse a simple piece of fruit or a salad of raw vegetables because they find them insipid.

Whoever has the will and the patience to stop using salt, in the first weeks will find that food is tasteless and it will be difficult to immediately appreciate the flavor. This is normal because our taste buds need time to regenerate. But, gradually, they will recover and enhance their innate sensitivity to flavors.

Another benefit that we get when we stop taking salt is that it allows the body to eliminate the old accumulations of toxic waste. This may temporarily cause some unpleasant symptoms such as headache, dark and abundant urine, burning during urination, irritation of the skin, mouth, eyes, etc. But it is actually a good sign. We just have to be patient and be happy because we are releasing numerous toxins.

Between the age of 30 and 40, and even before, there is usually a clogging of our hydraulic system. It is indeed the time when we begin to "fatten" (swelling) even if we eat less.

Many overweight people, if only they stopped eating salt, would lose several kilos in a short time because they would allow the body to significantly reduce the retention of water required to dilute salt. In a short time, depending on the individual's weight, from 5 to 20 kg of water can be lost. Being fat or swollen is not the same thing. Many people think they are fat when, in fact, they are simply swollen.

SALT IS BAD FOR THE HEART

According to the declaration of some Boston scholars in 2007, limiting our daily intake of salt reduces the risk of cardiovascular disease by 25 percent. Furthermore, the researchers argued that reducing salt intake lowers the mortality from cardiovascular disease. From 1990 till the present, scientists have tracked 5,000 people in order to identify the effects of salt on the human body.

The participants were divided into two groups: the first group ate normally; the second group ate food with less salt. This is the result so far: 70 percent of the first group had high blood pressure and, consequently, the risk of developing cardiovascular disease. But, only 200 people of the 2,500 in the second group (eight percent) had high blood pressure. The difference is remarkable: 1,800 persons in the first group compared to 200 in the second one.

Another interesting study is the one of Kacie M. Dickinson and his colleagues at the Commonwealth Scientific and Industrial Research Organization in Adelaide, Australia. The study tracked the health of 16 individuals, giving them a little salty tomato soup and, half an hour later, the same soup but ten times saltier.

The ultrasounds measured the amount of sodium present in the blood of the 16 members of the experimental group. It was found that the high concentration of salt in the arteries caused a narrowing of blood vessels. Let's see why.

When the heart pumps blood through the arteries, it produces a gas called nitrogen monoxide or nitrogen oxide, which relaxes arterial walls, makes the blood flow and promotes the oxygenation of the arteries, making them breathe and opening and restricting them if necessary. Scientists hypothesize that salt can cause malfunction of nitrogen oxide, hardening the arterial walls.

"The important aspect of this study," notes Sahil Parikh, interventional cardiologist at University Hospitals Case Medical Center and doctor of *AOL Health*, "is that it highlights that sodium has immediate and chronic effects on blood circulation."

Dr. Parikh reiterated as well that Dickinson's study is consistent with other studies, and that sodium-based diets should be discouraged because they are the cause of hypertension.

But salt is not only bad for the heart and kidneys, it can damage the brain too. This thesis is supported by a study carried out by the University of Toronto and published in the *Neurobiology of Aging* journal based on 1,262 healthy people, both men and women, between 67 and 84 years old.[93]

In accordance with this research, older people who keep a diet rich in salt show a quicker mental decline than those who are more careful in using the seasoning. The researchers arrived at these conclusions by examining once a year for three consecutive years the state of health of the subjects and using the most commonly used cognitive tests to diagnose Alzheimer's.

WHAT THE WHO SAYS

The World Health Organization has set a maximum amount of salt tolerated by an adult organism equal to five g per day. In fact, this is already a very high threshold since, according to the specialists, the

93 Fiocco, A. J., Shatenstein, B., et al., April 2012. *Sodium Intake and Physical Activity Impact Cognitive Maintenance in Older Adults: the NuAge Study.* Neurobiology of Aging. Volume 33, Issue 4.

correct amount for each of us should not exceed 600 mg of sodium per day. Athletes, however, need a little more.

Among processed products, the main source of salt in our diet is represented by the usual bread and bakery products—cookies, crackers, breadsticks, but also snacks, croissants, and cereal for breakfast. These are foods that commonly are not considered possible sources of salt but do contain more salt than we think.

In fact, cereal derivatives are a significant source of salt because they are consumed every day and in higher quantities than, for example, sausages, cheeses, canned fish, or chips, which contain the highest amounts of salt but are consumed in smaller quantities.

Even some condiments used in place of or in addition to salt are sodium-rich. This is the case, for example, of the bouillon cube (about 60 percent of it is made up of salt), also in the form of granules, of ketchup and soy sauce (14 percent). Other foods rich in salt are also ham (6.4 percent), cheese (4.5 percent), olives (3 percent), pickled vegetables (2.5 percent), and almost all industrial food.

A high consumption of salt is also associated with a higher risk of stomach cancer, increased urinary calcium losses and, thus, an increased risk of osteoporosis. Reducing the amount of salt we consume on a daily basis until its total elimination is not difficult, especially if the reduction occurs gradually.

In fact, our palates adapt easily and it is possible to reeducate it to foods without salt. Within a few months, or even weeks, those same foods will appear tasty at the right point. But those foods that we used to season will seem too salty.

Herbs and spices are a great alternative to salt and offer many advantages. They are rich in vitamins and minerals, stimulate digestion and facilitate purification.

From parsley to basil, from thyme to marjoram, from dandelion to red pepper, from saffron to curry, from nutmeg to ginger and cinnamon—we are just spoiled by plenty of choices. All of them flavor our dishes but without harmful side effects.

KATEMI

Katemi (1865–last available data 2010) is the name of an Indonesian woman who, like most of her fellow countrymen, has only one name. She was "discovered" by the National Institute of Statistics (BPS) commissioned to conduct the census of the population in Indonesia. The woman lived in the village of Bukit Batrem, in the province of Riau on the island of Sumatra.

When officials of the BPS visited her house in 2010, they could not believe they had an old woman in front of them. "Katemi had told us her year of birth, and when we calculated her age, we found that she was 145 years old," said Daryulis, one of the officials of the BPS.

To make sure it was not a mistake, the authorities deployed in the field a special team of agents. The person in charge of the investigation, Syafruddin, explained that he had done cross-checks to confirm the age of the woman who claimed to have been born in 1865. Eventually he was convinced that Katemi declared the truth. The team also interviewed some of her relatives and neighbors to see if they could confirm her statement.

"Katemi is the second of three children and was born in Wono Bondo, in the district of Pacitandi East Java, in 1865," said Ama, who claimed to be 98 years old and to be Katemi's younger sister.

Also Mimi (70 years old), Katemi's adopted daughter, reported to the team that she knew from Karyo, Katemi's brother, that her mother was born in 1865. According to the women, Karyo died in 2004 at the age of 165.

The information was confirmed as well by her grandchildren and great-grandchildren who declared that their grandmother liked to tell stories of her youth during the Portuguese, Dutch, and Japanese colonial eras.

Two neighbors of Katemi, Sutejo, aged 45, and Dwi, 50 years old, said that Katemi had lived in their village since 1980 and that over the years her face had not undergone significant changes.

"I think it is really possible that Katemi is 145 years old because she has a younger sister, who is 98 years old and a daughter who is more than 70 years old," said Dwi, one of Katemi's neighbors.

So if all the statements and investigations are true, then Katemi was born in the same year that Abraham Lincoln, the president of the United States, was killed, and when Lewis Carroll published for the first time *Alice in Wonderland*. It seems unbelievable, but it is true.

HER SECRET

It is said that life is like a soup. You get out of it what you put into it. No doubt, Katemi put into it the very best things: serenity, optimism, exercise, and a healthy nutrition.

Officially, we do not know the factors that have contributed to her longevity because of lack of research on it. However, as we have seen, all these centenarians have many features in common.

Albert Einstein said that the mind is like a parachute; it only works if you open it. Thus, if you want to live for a long time, you should open it.

SLIMMING AND DETOXIFYING TREATMENTS

Let us examine a topic that we mentioned in the section "Pills, Elixir of Long Life," namely, slimming and detoxifying treatments.

We will see how the self-styled experts and inventors of miraculous cures or amazing slimming treatments exploit the common childhood fantasy of magic pills, creams, massages, and more. As we have seen, there is something for everyone: the cream that slims the belly while we sleep; the pill that promises to burn kilos of fat while we are resting; the electric shock that makes us thin and toned without moving from our couch; the tonic for all seasons; the massage that degreases and relaxes.

To give credibility to these magical promises of modern sorcerers, the promises are attached to concepts such as magnetism, oxygen, water, energy, retention, drainage, and toxins. All these concepts fall within the cultural repertoire of a diploma but are manipulated and distorted for the use and consumption of the industry of miracles.

The trick is to borrow from physiology the functions of a molecule and pass off the sensational new discovery of hot water. They instill in us the idea that if a molecule is involved in the metabolism of fats then, we are all deficient in it and the principle of the quantity applies: the more you take, the more fat you burn.

But this is not the case. The more I take, the more I risk intoxication, creating very serious damage, as in the case of iron-based supplements which are sold as a panacea for all ills. The same applies to other minerals, vitamins, proteins, and seaweed slimming. Let us look at the main scientific legend.

DETOX WATER . . . ALIAS RUST WEIGHT IN GOLD

In 2002, in England, a footbath detox called "foot detox" had a high resonant advertising, according to which the device would allow the expulsion of toxins from our body through the feet. This equipment has been reproduced by many other companies with different names while maintaining the unique characteristics of the "ancestor" device. Today we find it especially in health centers under the names: Aqua Detox, Bio Detox, or Foot Detox.

How does it work? In practice, you plunge your feet into a pan full of water with some salts that is connected to an electrode. After 30 minutes, the session ends and the water magically takes on a generally brownish coloration.

What does this sensational device do? Here is what its inventor says: "Plunging the feet in warm water containing natural organic salts, with a slight current that resonates with your bioenergetic field passing through it, will encourage the expulsion of toxins from the 2,000 pores present in our feet." So the color of the water at the end of the session would be justified by the expulsion of toxins through our feet.

But this "godsend" was over in 2004 when Dr. Ben Goldacre revealed in the pages of the newspaper *The Guardian* what lies behind the much-vaunted wonder.[94] Being sure of the fraudulent nature of the device, the doctor wanted to do some tests to clear up any doubts.

For the first experiment he used a bowl with water and salt, and two nails attached to a car battery. As if by magic, the water took on the same color as the one obtained at the end of a session with the "foot detox."

For the second experiment, he sent a friend of his, Dr. Mark Atkins, to undergo the treatment with the device. In both cases, a sample of water was taken at the beginning and at the end of the session.

The samples were then sent for analysis to the Medical Toxicology Unit of New Cross, which, without any amazement for Goldacre, reported the following results: before the treatment, the water contained 0.54 mg of iron per liter. After the treatment, it contained 23.6 mg/l. The water of the experiment with the nails contained 97 mg/l and was, in fact, darker.

Basically, the device produced rust. It was nothing more than

---

94 Ben Goldacre, "Rusty results," *The Guardian*, September 2, 2004.

the rust produced by the corrosion of the electrodes, and this is the only reason for the color of the water. Furthermore, the color change occurred in any case, whether or not the feet were immersed.

Ultimately, the skin has no ability to excrete toxins. The real detoxification of foreign substances occurs in the liver. In fact, the liver changes foreign substances' chemical structure so that the kidneys, which later filter them from the blood to the urine, can excrete them.

"Basically, the manufacturers of these devices provide a dialysis through the feet. Urea and creatinine are probably the smallest molecules—if you prefer, you can call them toxins—which the body excretes through urine and sweat. If some toxins went out, they would be present too. Instead, in the water there was no trace of toxins either before or after the treatment," says Dr. Goldacre.

This equipment is sold at a price that ranges from $200 to $3,500, and the "treatment" in a beauty center costs around $50 for a 30-minute session.

This is an example in which science is used to foster the popular credulity and the portfolio of pseudo-healers. The equipment used for detoxification is therefore a scam in all respects, and at the end of the treatment the person treated will have only a little rust on her feet.

AND WHAT ABOUT SWEAT?

Sweat, in spite of the popular belief that considers it a vehicle of massive amounts of "toxins," consists of 99 percent water and, in that tiny one percent that remains, we find urea, creatinine, ammonia, mineral salts, and some medication if consumed.

With regard to the minerals lost with sweating, we should not spend money on supplements, since they are compensated without problems through nutrition. For example, the calcium, magnesium, and potassium lost with three liters of sweat are reinstated with a glass of tomato juice or orange juice. And losing three liters of sweat is not so common, if we think that in the 90 minutes of a football game a player loses about two liters.

The sweat excretes waste matter, but in an incidental and quantitatively insignificant amount compared to feces and urine. Its main function is thermoregulation: by evaporating, it subtracts energy from the body compensating for the discomfort caused by the high temperatures generated by physical effort.

So sweat plays a fundamental role, but only in the context of the regulation of our body temperature. Nothing more. Let us not give sweat a dignity which it does not have in reality. Entrusting the elimination of waste substances to sweat means to entrust the cleaning of the house to ants: they will take away only the crumbs.

THE SAUNA AND THE TURKISH BATH

We saw that sweat is just a lot of water; it corresponds to a very small fraction of the volume of the metabolic waste and few salts. Nothing more. So we give to the sauna and the Turkish bath the pleasure of relaxing without thinking of delirious dreams of "detoxification."

DO NOT MIX UP SWEAT AND FAT

Some beauty farms adopt the cunning strategy of making the unaware customer do physical activity in a warm/humid environment, or under the bombardment of infrared light, in order to dissolve fat. They do nothing but increase sweating.

Measurements of body weight, waist, or thigh circumference, are made before and after the physical activity. The results are always amazing. Why? Because the client, after just one session of "slimming treatment," is left with a few centimeters less on the waist, hips, or thigh. But what has the client actually lost?

He has lost water. Can that person really declare victory? Two or three sessions more and they can go to the beach without any weight or cellulite problems? It does not work that way. The apprentice sorcerers of these looting pecuniary beauty centers know this very well.

Just to give an example, after running five km, a person who weighs 66 kg will lose only 16.5 grams of fat.[95] Those who tried to run five km know that they are not just a few kilometers, especially if the person is not trained. Exhausted and out of breath, after a run of this magnitude one could imagine that he burned loads and loads of fat, and the scales seem to confirm this way of thinking: one kg less than before the race. However, if we analyze this kilo of organic material, things change: there are 983.5 grams of sweat against only 16.5 grams of fat. So in order to lose, let us say, one kg of fat, we would have to run 303 km; 1,000 gr / 16,5 × 5 km = 303 km.

I would say that we are a very low-cost car, considering that with one kg of fuel (fat) a person of 66 kg can do 303 km. Not even the lightest car in the world, the Peel P50, which weighs only 59 kg,

---

95 In the chapter "Physical Activity," in the second volume, we will see how to calculate, based on weight and the km run, both the calories and the fat loss, either during a normal walk or during a race.

does more than 50 kilometers with a liter of gas.

In the next volume we will discuss how to really get rid of body fat and how to calculate our ideal weight.

THE TRICK OF HIGH-PROTEIN DIETS

Another trick aimed at losing water and muscle mass, namely the one that is responsible for the elimination of fat and calories, is the high-protein diet.

In practice, we have to give up carbohydrates in the name of proteins and, instead of them, start eating meat, cold cuts, and fish in abundance—perhaps starting with a week based on fruit and vegetables.

Nevertheless, the elimination of carbohydrates in favor of a surplus of proteins leads to consuming our stock of carbohydrates stored in the muscles and liver that amounts to about 500 grams. What does it mean?

It is known that one gram of carbohydrates holds about 3.5 grams of water in the body. Therefore, together with the stock of 500 grams of carbohydrates "burned" for the failure to introduce sugar in the diet, we also lose automatically 1.75 kg of water, namely: 500 × 3.5 = 1.750 grams of water, plus the 500 grams of carbohydrates.

Since carbohydrate fasting leads the body to consume the stocks within 24/48 hours, at the end, after two days, we will have lost 2.25 kg of water. The unaware victim of the wrong diet will be thrilled with the outcome. The subject will wrongly translate this result as a fat loss. Actually, the fat will be stored at the expense of the muscles!

The consequences?

- Loss of muscle—it is equivalent to a slower and slower metabolism.
- Loss of water—it means affecting the functionality of the muscles, including their function of fat disposal.
- The muscle protein "burned" to replace the sugars produces large amounts of nitrogen, ammonia, and urea, which decalcify bones and teeth, overload kidneys and liver, and acidify the blood. Thus, we lose additional water through the urine to dispose of these waste products.
- Alteration of the acid-based equilibrium.

LOSING WEIGHT THROUGH FASTING

Fasting is a powerful tool that should be used with caution since it is a double-edged sword. If we do not know how to use it, it is likely to do more harm than good. To this topic will be dedicated an entire chapter in the next volume. For the moment, suffice it to say that if used well, fasting prolongs life, cures cancer and many other serious diseases.

DIET PILLS

Diet pills are divided into two categories: drugs and supplements. In the first case, slimming tablets are sold only in pharmacies, usually with a medical prescription. Instead, in the second case, the tables for weight loss are available to everyone. We can find them in supplements shops, in supermarkets, health food stores, on the Internet, and in pharmacies.

Before going any further, let us clear up a basic concept: the magic pill that makes us lose weight does not exist.

The American FDA (Food and Drug Administration) warns and explains, "Slimming pills and dietary supplements do not exist. We must be wary of the advertisements that promise all this. But above all, we must pay attention to what is contained in the tablets or herbal teas often passed off as 'natural.'"

So, regardless of the diet and physical exercise, there is nothing that is able to make us lose body fat without harming our health or without producing important imbalances. Anyone who promises something like that lies.

The desire to lose weight, the need to improve both our aesthetics and our health, are often found in laziness, lack of will, in depression, or simply in the lack of time or the ability to manage ourselves, an obstacle that often seems insurmountable. Unfortunately, this desire revolves around perhaps the biggest scam that has ever been made in the field of medicine.

Let us start with diet drugs. What are they? How do they work? Are they dangerous?

They are divided into two categories:

a) Anorectics (substances that reduce the feeling of hunger);
b) Lipase inhibitors (substances that block the absorption of lipids in the intestine).

Weight-loss drugs are the ones that really make us slim. However, they are also the ones causing more side effects and are used not for overweight people, but only for truly obese people. What does this mean?

It means that these drugs are reserved only for those patients for whom obesity is a risk factor that is much higher than the medications. In a nutshell, between the two evils, choose the lesser. Since these people are likely to die at any time because of a cardiac arrest, doctors choose the "less dangerous" way and prescribe the pills.

Let us see what are the side effects of weight-loss drugs: death, stroke, heart disease, valvular heart injury, addiction, depression, states of hyperarousal, uncontrolled anxiety, tremor, insomnia, nervousness, psychosis, suicidal thoughts, tachycardia, palpitation, memory loss, risk of deformation for newborns, high blood pressure, digestive disorders, severe intestinal diseases, flatulence, incontinence, just to name a few.

And here is the cherry on top: When we stop taking the medicine, which must not be taken for more than three months, the appetite returns even more intensely, causing the immediate recovery of the kilos that were lost.

At this point, it is clear what all these people face. In order to lose a few kilos, maybe because they are slightly overweight or, even worse, because of an aesthetics factor, people buy these drugs on the black market or on the Internet. Recall that only obese people can buy them and only through a medical prescription.

In these cases, a balanced diet and regular exercise are the best treatments. There are no magic pills to lose weight, or at least not without serious risks to a person's health. And what about food supplements?

They too, are divided into two categories:

a)   Those that replicate the effects of anorectic drugs;
b)   Those that are rich in fiber.

Michael Levy, head of the division for new drugs and labels complying with the FDA, on the government website explains:

"These products are not legal dietary supplements. They are actually very powerful drugs masquerading as natural or 'herbal' products. They involve significant risks to unaware consumers. In fact, there have been cases of deaths due to the use of these weight-loss products. In some of them, sold as dietary supplements, we found dangerous hidden ingredients, including banned drugs, others for blood pressure, and still others that are not approved in the United States."

Remember the Swiss Institute study on therapeutic products? In the laboratory, after analyzing 122 samples of "diet pills" that are all the rage on the Internet, it was discovered that nine out of 10 contain harmful substances. Moreover, one-third of the packs, although declared as purely herbal, contained chemical ingredients.

The risk, of course, is not about all the supplements for weight loss. It is necessary to distinguish and be sure that there are no side effects. Even when they go well, these supplements are just a waste of money. For example, look at those supplements that use dietary fiber that, taken together with generous amounts of water, swell within the stomach, offering the feeling of satiety. It is a hundred times more healthy and cheaper to eat fresh fruits and vegetables than ingesting these supplements.

Another example is constituted by the thermogenic ones that determine the increase in metabolic activity of the body, raising its temperature and increasing the heartbeat. There are plenty of them. The principal ingredients can be extracts of bitter orange, cocoa, coffee, guarana, mate, black tea, and green tea. We have already seen how caffeine from coffee and tea activates our metabolism. Remember the example of the whip and the horse. All the whips (stimulators) are to be avoided. It is interesting to note that in order to live longer, we have to have a slower heartbeat and a lower temperature, the exact opposite of what thermogenic supplements do. A slow heartbeat can be reached by following a diet based on raw vegetables, or by physical activity, it is not possible to lower body temperature without dying. Some Russian researchers discovered that if we could lower the internal temperature by only 2°C, we could easily live up to 200 years.

Another thing that unites all weight-loss supplements, but also the entire weight-loss industry, is the misleading advertising. The number of penalties for misleading advertising is indeed very vast. Every country has, or at least should have, an authority with the task of protecting the consumer, prohibiting and punishing unfair trade practices, unfair contract terms, and misleading advertising.

To give an example, let us go to the Italian website of the AGCM (in Italian Autorità Garante della Concorrenza e del Mercato), better known as the Antitrust Authority, under the section "measures." (The undertaken measures are in Italian only, as they relate to Italian advertising.)

To get there, just go to the website—www.agcm.it—click on the top right on "Search," then "Advanced search measures," and then check "Consumer Protection." Without changing anything, we type into the "Search" box the word that we are interested in.

So, for example, today, (August 5, 2012), as I write these lines, if I type the word cellulite, I find 213 results. Almost all these cases are resolved with convictions for misleading advertising. And that is just for the anti-cellulite products. This list is constantly growing, and maybe in a year instead of 213 results we will find 230 or even more.

If I type:

1. *Anti-wrinkle creams* – 459 results
2. *Belly cream* – 471 results
3. *Weight loss* – 811 results
4. *Face cream* – 2,727 results

Below, I will only list some penalties for misleading advertising of the most popular brands and products. I think this may already offer a solid evidence of bad faith. However, if we want to know more about the matter, we can check the resolution in which we are interested, and on the document in PDF format we will find all the scientific reasons for which the product does not meet the boasted requirements that led to the conviction. So, let us take this step by step.

For example, in Italy, who has never heard of the weight-loss supplements "Giorno & Notte"? They are advertised practically all hours of the day, and the children as soon as they hear the publicity tune sing it because they already know it by heart. Consider that years ago my sister bought them as well. Here is the measure:

PI5813 – AMERICAN DIET SYSTEM GIORNO E NOTTE
Measure No. 17811
December 27, 2007

The Antitrust Authority claims that the advertisements in issue are likely to mislead consumers with regard to the actual features of the slimming products advertised, as well as with regard to how to benefit from the guarantee of repayment of the price paid promised in advertisements in question . . . also, that these advertisements are liable to endanger the health and safety of consumers . . . causing them to disregard the normal rules of prudence and vigilance, in particular physiological and pathological conditions.

The fine: **80,000 Euros**

Another weight loss supplement is Kilocal. Let us see the corresponding measure:

PS1898 – POOL PHARMA-KILOCAL
Measure No. 21539
September 8, 2010

The Authority considered that the commercial practice in question is incorrect in that it is likely to mislead people about the real characteristics of the product and likely to affect the economic behavior of consumers, causing them to purchase the advertised product on the basis of an erroneous perception of its real nature as well as its potentialities. With the advertisements in question, disseminated via the Internet, the press, television, and radio, the professional intends to communicate to the potential buyers the idea that the product would be able to carry out an inhibitory action in the assimilation of excess fat. In this regard, the frequent use of words evocative of a practical, safe, and innovative remedy against the absorption of calories, associated with the image of dishes and desserts as an accompaniment to slogans such as "Don't give up the pleasure of eating," have a high persuasive value to the average consumer. The latter, in fact, is inclined to think that the mere use of the product in question is enough to solve a problem such as the increase in body weight due to a high-calorie diet. In this respect, the explicit indication of the pharmacy as a channel of purchase strengthens its position in the consumer opinion on the reliability and effectiveness of the product. Also, the use of scientific terminology, with terms borrowed from the world of chemistry, pharmaceutics, and also the processes involved in human anatomy to describe the composition and the phases of the assimilation of the product.

The fine: **200,000 Euros**

Since we are talking about well-being, let us take a look at other health products. We can start from the cute silicone bracelet, the *Power Balance*. Here is what its producer says:

"Power Balance is the most advanced energy system available in the world today. It is a natural amplifier of energy that immediately tunes your body to have great performance. Increase of resistance, strength, body balance, flexibility... an energy system, a natural amplifier of energy, which by entering in resonance with the chemical and biological increases its efficiency instantaneously... suitable for any type of sport... reduces stress, chronic pain, carsickness, seasickness and many other ailments... designed to increase body balance, coordination, strength, flexibility and endurance."

Here is the measure:

PS6307 – POWER BALANCE- SILICONE BRACELET
Measure No. 21956
December 22, 2010

The Antitrust Authority says that there is no scientific evidence that can support what is being advertised as well as any contraindications associated with the use of the bracelet. As a result, the advertising messages of the "Power Balance" must be considered misleading. With regard to the actual subject, the challenged business practice, questioned by the professionals, consists in having attributed to the neoprene and silicone bracelets, as well as the necklaces branded "Power Balance," qualities, properties, and effects on body balance, strength, and physical resistance, which are not true.

The fine: **350,000 Euros**

Probably we have all seen the lies about wrinkles, cellulite and fat? Here are some examples:

1. Liftactiv Retinol HA (Vichy)
2. Vital Restore (Garnier)
3. Cellu-metric (Vichy)
4. Ultralift (Garnier)
5. Rimodel Collagene (l'Oreal)

Here is what the slogans of these products say: "Against all types of wrinkles: permanent, reversible, embryonic." "The treatment is able to fill the permanent wrinkles in a month" (thanks to the retinol and hyaluronic acid), with the ability to "stimulate the cell viability also of mature skin." "80% of its users can notice a reduction of dark spots," ". . . smoothing out of the skin, fat relocation and losing of centimeters," "... . . breaking down fat deposits and stretching the orange peel skin; night action: it relocates fats and prevents restocking." "It stretches the skin in an hour, reduces wrinkles, even marked ones, in just 15 days." "In an hour, it stretches the skin by 83%." "In 15 days it reduces wrinkles by 78%."

The following is the respective measure:

PS4030 – VICHY-L'ORÉAL-GARNIER
Measure No. 20862
March 3, 2010

After an endless series of investigations, the Antitrust Authority fined the mother company, L'Oreal, for misleading advertising. For more information, see the document including the measure that consists of 18 pages.

The fine: **270,000 Euros**

As we can see, there is no magic cream (not even L'Oreal has it) that can reduce or eliminate wrinkles, cellulite, or fat. There are hundreds of antifat-cellulite-wrinkle products. If even one of them worked, it would deserve the Nobel Prize and the monopoly of the market. Unfortunately, there is none. If it really existed, people would not have any more wrinkles or cellulite and would no longer be overweight or obese.

On the Internet, there are numerous "health" products, such as pills, elixirs, bracelets, earrings, magnets, talismans, and creams that promise everything and do nothing. Be wary of those who tell us that thanks to their product we will feel better, stronger, and so on. They are all crooks. We do not live in a world of fairy tales where there are supernatural powers and magic potions.

Be wary also of all the magicians and sorcerers who promise to predict the future or to solve our problems. They are all lies. No one can do that! The only real magic that is available in this world is information. Information is what made me realize that in order to live as long as possible, to stay young and beautiful as long as possible, not to get sick, never to get fat, etc., one must follow the rules that I have written in this volume and will write in future ones. After internalizing the full knowledge and the awareness of these books, you will get everything you want from your life.

I am referring to the fact that it all starts with health. When you are really healthy, everything else comes by itself. Also, our mind thinks differently. And it is even easier to become rich. Believing is seeing.

One last thing: Electrostimulators, contrary to popular belief, do not make us lose weight; they do not sculpt the abdomen, thighs, and buttocks. The same thing applies to vibrating platforms as well. It is not true that they make us strong, thin, and toned. There are two more lies that I am not going to debunk, otherwise I run the risk of going into too much detail. If someone is interested in further investigating this topic, he or she can check on the Internet and do all the necessary research.

For the moment, the important thing is to know that these tools not only do not do anything of what they promise, but are even detrimental to our health.

In the Next Volume

Dear reader, I am absolutely sure that you have found a real treasure in this book and that you will find other treasures in the next volumes. As you may have noticed, the reasoning of this series of volumes goes in one direction. Why? Think about health and disease. What do you notice? It is about two things that are absolutely opposed.

You can have one or the other. You cannot have both of them. As Jesus said: "Whoever is not with me is against me." Well, the same goes for your health. Everything that does not go toward health, goes toward the disease.

Logic tells us that two opposite things cannot go in the same direction. But this is precisely what modern medicine tries to do. And it is not because it does not know but because it is in its interest. The reason is profit. Let me give you one example to illustrate this point.

Let us take salt as an example. We already saw that it can only harm us, whether it is table salt, unrefined, or sea salt. Therefore, where will it lead us? Does it lead us toward health or toward the disease? Toward the disease, it is obvious. And a lesser consumption of salt does not mean that it is good for our health. It will affect my health less, that is all. However, in both cases it is bad. It does not matter if the punch you take in your face is strong or not; it will hurt you in both cases. It does not matter if the knife with which a person is stabbed is long or short; it will hurt either way.

The key feature of this book—and of the next ones—is exactly this. It has no middle ground, because it does not exist. Telling lies is needless. If something harms our health, it harms it and that is that. It must be said, and then it is up to the readers to decide whether or not to harm their health by themselves. But at least they have the opportunity to make an informed choice. Unfortunately, this possibility today is no longer found in any book.

Many people are willing to follow any diet as long as it is effective. The problem is that 99 percent of them are the result of pure imagination.

Just think about the fact that there is a modern writer who published a book in which he says that we should eat our feces spread on a slice of raw meat. And there are people who tried it!

In the next volume we will resume our journey into the realm of health and we will have 10 more chapters that are fundamental to our well-being and life lengthening.

In the chapter, "White Bread," we will talk about refined foods and how white flour and its derivatives are a major cause of disease. We will also take into consideration how white bread is deprived of all its nutrients and transformed into an empty food, a dead food, and without life energy.

Another chapter will be dedicated to fat: "Fats and Energy." In this chapter, we will shed light on a much debated topic: Are fats good or bad? We will also talk about bioenergy and how those calories should not be seen as a tool for measuring the biological value.

"Physical Activity" will be a chapter full of useful information—

how much and how to train properly. The dream of many parents is to see their children becoming professional athletes. But did you know that statistically an athlete lives a shorter life than any other professional?

One of the chapters that you should absolutely not miss is the one about "The Power of the Mind." If you can control your mind, you can control your life too. We will talk about the mysterious forces of the mind and how to control them. We will then see how life is nothing but the result of our thoughts and how to pay attention to what we believe possible, namely to our beliefs—or convictions—because they determine what we do and, therefore, the results we get.

After that we have the chapter "Medicinal Herbs." Can they extend life or are they actually overvalued? How can we use them correctly? What are they and when should we use them? All these questions, and many other questions, will be answered in this chapter.

In the chapter "Drugs or Poisons?" we will see where medical progress is actually selling diseases. The American Cancer Society (ACS) reports that 47 percent of men and 38 percent of women will get cancer during their lifetime. One out of four of these people will die prematurely of cancer. A brief chapter is dedicated to this great problem.

Another important chapter will be "Inheritance." Cancer, diabetes, and obesity are not hereditary. Neither are predispositions to disease. Life is controlled by the environment and not by genes. Genes are only the programs that are activated or deactivated by the environment in which we live. The genetic inheritance is a hoax of modern medicine.

We will also talk about tea, soft drinks, and energizing drinks in the chapter "Drinks that Harm Your Health Are Bad." How and why are they dangerous? This is a chapter that will clarify once and for all why they should be avoided.

The chapter on "Fasting" will tell us how and when to use it. Through this tool many nutritionists, including Hippocrates, took care of their patients with diabetes, cancer, and other diseases. Even Jesus practiced it and handed it down to his disciples. The beliefs of many religions still keep practicing fasting.

Finally, in the last chapter, "Body Hygiene," we will see how the shampoos, soaps, and toothpastes, apart from being useless, are also very toxic to our bodies. We will see how you can wash your hair, body, and teeth without these chemical poisons. Did you know that hair falls out mainly because of shampoo? And did you know that the toxic substances in these cleaners migrate and settle day after day in your body?

Space will be dedicated to the lives of long-living people and the myths and realities of health.

Further on, we will talk about how and what to eat. At the end of this course, when you have assimilated all the knowledge you need, we will talk about diet and recipes. You cannot help a person drive a Ferrari before teaching him how to drive.

I will wait for you in the next volume! See you soon.

Sergiu Damian